Praise for *Coloring Outside the Lines*

In Coloring Outside the Lines, Jan Adrian empowers readers with her wonderful wisdom, learned by navigating a life of ongoing challenges and chronic cancer. She teaches us the power of following our own unique path, trusting our intuition, and finding our courage and grounding through friendships and spirituality.

~ Sandra Marinella, author of

The Story You Need to Tell—Writing to Heal from Trauma, Illness, or Loss

Jan Adrian founded a non-profit group called *Healing Journeys.* She learned to co-journey with cancer and used her cancer experience as a turning point in her life—which is why she is telling her story more than thirty years after her first encounter with multiple relapsing breast cancer. The greatest enemy of anyone with cancer is fear. Reading Jan's healing story, you will understand how she transcended fear. The details of every person who has encountered cancer in their body and reached a healing/healthy state, differ from one and other. However, the underlying principles are very similar. There isn't a "magic bullet" for cancer. There is however, a magic matrix. Learn how Jan found her magic matrix.

~ Dwight L. McKee,
MD, CNS, ABIHM, Board certified in Medical Oncology

There are many books on the subject of cancer and the personal journeys that people go on in response to the diagnosis. But rarely is a book written with the emphasis on living with cancer and not fighting with it. Indeed, I think the wisdom in this approach is profoundly needed by all of us, since, in fact, we are all threatened by mortality in one way or another. As Jan writes, "the trick is not to let finite events eclipse the infinite." The book is an expression of a deeper truth, one that has taken courage and conviction to attain, and clarity of purpose to be able to share in a way that will produce the desired effect in the reader – inspiration. We can all be grateful that there are people like Jan who show us the way, heroes among us, pointing out the hidden blessings in each challenge that we face while alive. Jan teaches us that while living and surviving are important, to thrive is our greater potential that is achievable when we resist being restricted by fear. This requires that we evolve in our thinking and response to discomfort. In that respect, this book is a gift that will help you find your own way.

~ Michael Finkelstein, MD, author of
Slow Medicine: Hope and Healing for Chronic Illness

Jan is an expert at coloring outside the lines and this skill has proven time and again to be the reason she is still here teaching and inspiring the rest of us to do the same. Her vulnerability in offering up this memoir helps folks realize how deeply biography impacts biology.

~ Nasha Winters, ND, FABNO

Jan Adrian has been living with recurrent breast cancer for more than 30 years and with stage 4 cancer for 11 of those years. Her life story – especially how she managed her diagnosis, treatments, recurrences, and "outside the lines" integrative therapies – will inspire anyone touched by cancer. Jan shows us how it's possible to thrive with cancer, and how cancer can be managed all while living a full, robust life.

~ Kelly A. Turner, PhD, NY Times Bestselling author of
Radical Hope and *Radical Remission*

After a lifetime of navigating illness while staying vital, Jan Adrian offers much hard-earned wisdom in her brave and honest memoir, *Coloring Outside the Lines*. Jan is a wise and steadfast guide who never fails to penetrate trouble for the life-giving medicine at its center. This book will be a huge help to others.

~ Mark Nepo, author of
Surviving Storms and *The Book of Awakening*

COLORING
outside the lines

COLORING
outside the lines

Surviving and Thriving
with Cancer for 30+ Years

a memoir by
JAN ADRIAN

For permission please contact:
Jan Adrian
EMAIL jan@healingjourneys.org
ADDRESS PO Box 221417 • Sacramento, CA 95822

Coloring Outside the Lines, Surviving and Thriving with Cancer for 30+ Years
Published by Pretzel Paws Press

Library of Congress Control Number: 2023911971

ISBN 979-8-9880221-0-7

Copyright language: English

Printed by IngramSpark, Publishers Group West
Berkeley, California USA

Dedicated to the Spirit Alive in Each of Us

TABLE OF CONTENTS

FOREWORD by Terri Tate
INTRODUCTION: Both - And

PART ONE: DEFINING MOMENTS

PART TWO: EARLY STEPPING STONES

PART THREE: LATER BUILDING BLOCKS

PART FOUR: TURNING POINTS

PART FIVE: STRATEGIES FOR MANAGING CANCER

EPILOGUE

GRATITUDE & RESOURCES

Foreword and Introduction

FOREWORD

"I'm not even sure I want to write a memoir."

Jan and I are sitting on my beige leather living room couch.

She is in town to participate in my first ever memoir writing class which will be held in this room the next day.

"But you have such an amazing story to tell. Think of all the people you can help."

I had told Jan's story countless times in the two-plus decades I'd known her. Everyone who heard it was inspired beyond measure, not only because she had been living with cancer for such a long time, but because hers is a meaningful, vibrant life, and she had encouraged thousands of people.

"And you have such a great title."

A few months earlier, Jan had sat on this same couch to take part in a storytelling class where she told of her traumatic experience with self-expressive coloring (Chapter 1). She concluded with, "And I've been coloring outside the lines ever since."

We agreed that this was her title if she ever decided to write a memoir.

Three years later, almost to the day, Jan called to ask if I would write the foreword to this book. It had taken me twenty years to write my memoir, so I had to get by my jealousy, but this was Jan. When she sets her mind to something, you don't want to be in her way, even if you are cancer.

When Jan was first diagnosed with breast cancer in 1989, she found the standard medical approach wanting when it came to her emotional, spiritual and nutritional needs. Never one to sit around and whine about a problem, Jan set out to solve it. She created *Cancer as a Turning Point, From Surviving to Thriving*™ conferences to fill that gap and has helped more than 25,000 people at thirty-seven gatherings since then.

I had the honor to speak at an early conference and became part of the Healing Journeys family. Cancer patients and their loved ones received an exquisite blend of inspiration, education and support. Jan ran these amazing events with military precision and an open heart.

Jan has co-habitated with cancer for three decades and has lived a full, fun and meaningful life. You are lucky to get to read about it. In these pages you will find inspiration to create that kind of life for yourself. Regardless of the kind of challenges you may face, Jan's story will support you whenever you, too, want to color outside the lines.

Terri Tate, RN, MS
December 2022
Humorist, Author & Memoir Mentor

INTRODUCTION
Both - And

This is a cancer memoir, but it's not a story of how I became cancer free, because I didn't. My first cancer diagnosis was in 1989. I've had three primary cancers—breast cancer in both breasts and ocular melanoma—and more recurrences than I can count. I've had breast cancer metastasized to my lungs since 2011. Essentially, cancer has been a chronic illness for me for over thirty years. My story is about living fully and thriving with cancer.

Most people see cancer as a death sentence, and the primary reaction is fear. Once they receive a diagnosis, they want to eradicate every cancer cell from their body, and they live in constant fear of a recurrence. Their focus is on fighting the cancer, attacking the tumor, trying to kill the intruder. There is another way to address cancer that may involve more curiosity than fear.

We all have cancer cells in our bodies at some time. Our immune systems are meant to eliminate them. We don't need to get rid of every cancer cell to live a happy full life, but we do need to keep cancer from progressing. My focus has been on creating a terrain in the body that isn't conducive to the growth of cancer, and that also stimulates the self-healing mechanism of the body, as it was designed.

These two methods of dealing with cancer don't pose an either/or question. It's a both/and. There is both fear and curiosity. And there is both fighting the tumor and supporting the self-healing ability of the body.

I don't definitively know why I'm still alive after more than thirty years of living with cancer. *Coloring Outside the Lines* describes in detail what I've done, both to create the bodily environment that doesn't contribute to cancer's growth, and to eliminate tumors. I haven't been a passive consumer of cancer treatments; I've been involved in choosing and implementing my treatments. I've sought second opinions, looked at the research, trusted my intuition and decided what the best course of action was for me. I haven't always done what the doctor recommended. I've said yes to medical treatments when the benefit was greater than the risk, or when the treatment wouldn't diminish my quality of life. With every medically recommended treatment, I've asked about the research behind the treatment and how much that treatment would benefit me. If the answer was a 5% benefit with severe damaging side effects, I didn't embrace the treatment. If it was a 97% benefit with very few side effects, undertaking the treatment was a no-brainer.

Over my thirty-plus years living with cancer, I've engaged in allopathic (Western mainstream medicine); alternative healing methods (Nutrition and Three V's); Radical Remission strategies (Social Support); cutting edge treatments (Proton Beam Radiation and Cryoablation)— as well as treatments used as a matter of protocol in Europe (Mistletoe), but virtually unknown in the U.S. You'll see that in Part Five, "Strategies for Managing Cancer," I elaborate on these treatments and my physical, mental and spiritual reactions to each of them.

My main focus has been on giving my mind, body and soul what it needs for self-healing. I believe in the self-healing mechanism of the body. I see it in action any time I cut my finger and watch it heal without my conscious aid. I experienced it when I was sixteen and had an illness that couldn't be diagnosed, thus couldn't be treated by the medical profession. Once we gave my body the nutrients it needed, healing took place without medical treatment. This belief has allowed me to make cancer treatment decisions not based on fear, but on a trust in my body.

The question I've most frequently been asked by other people touched by cancer is, "How do you remain calm and not panic in the face of a cancer recurrence?" In this book, I address this question by describing the beliefs and attitudes that have facilitated me through eighty years of life and more than thirty years of living with cancer. In my childhood home, there was a plaque on the wall with a Bible verse that read, "All things work together for good" (Romans 8:28). Even though I've moved on from the religion of my childhood, I still choose to believe that message. When something happens that can be interpreted as bad or negative, if I look more deeply, I can usually find gifts, or something good in the experience. When a cancer recurrence appeared, I usually started out with an immediate "Oh, Shit" reaction, but eventually I was able to look for the silver lining.

I've never met anyone whose immediate response to a diagnosis of cancer is, "Thank you for this gift." It's not something I would have chosen, yet I've heard people say cancer is a gift. For many survivors, their life after cancer is better than their life before cancer. If you have lost a loved one from cancer or if you have experienced the fear of a cancer diagnosis, this may seem counter-intuitive or even impossible. But if you are living with a cancer diagnosis, it may be an idea worth exploring.

Were there hidden blessings in cancer for me? My cancer diagnosis started me on a new career that has given me great satisfaction for over twenty-five years. And many of the people I treasure in my life now wouldn't be in my circle of friends if it weren't for cancer. Because of the changes I've made in my life in response to the cancer diagnosis, I may be healthier now than before I was diagnosed with cancer. Cancer has been a motivator for me to improve my diet, use guided imagery, meditate, reduce stress, look for joy, let go of negative emotions, trust my intuition, identify and embrace my purpose in living, and practice gratitude. I think this has all contributed to the evolution of my soul, in addition to my thriving in this life.

Sometimes the benefits of a situation are not obvious with my limited vision on the earthly plane, so another attitude I embrace is that *I am a Spiritual being on a human path*. Spirit outlives matter. Everything that happens to me in this earth school is for the purpose of growing my soul. After my initial emotional reaction, I try not to label any event as good or bad. Events in my life don't happen to me. They happen for me. Often the gifts in what could be called a negative situation have promoted the growth of my soul.

I was devastated when I was diagnosed with breast cancer in 1989 at age forty-seven. My life up to that point had taught me to be curious, intuitive, to trust Divine guidance, and to color outside the lines. Most of the stories in this book are about specific events in my life that helped to form or strengthen the attitudes, beliefs, and lifestyle that have been major resources in supporting me through more than thirty years of thriving with cancer. Something I've done to manage my cancers has made a difference, but I can't be sure what. Even if I knew, I couldn't tell you what would make a difference for you. This isn't a "how-to" book. We're unique individuals and we each need to figure out what's best for us. My wish is that hearing my story will create hope and other options for the millions of people who think cancer, especially a recurrence, is a death sentence. My hope is that those who hear my story will be curious and discover in its pages something that might be of assistance in learning to thrive with whatever has washed up on your beach.

Defining Moments

CHAPTER ONE

Coloring Outside the Lines

I'M IN A COLD, STERILE room with a large piece of equipment. Extending out from the equipment is a narrow platform on which the technician asks me to lie down on my back. She covers me with a warm blanket, puts a pillow under my knees to protect my back, and supports my arms so they won't fall off the platform. I ask her if it matters if my arms are by my side or on my stomach. She says it doesn't matter as long as I don't move them. I am having a PET/CT scan to see what's going on in my body because my quarterly cancer marker number has just gone up considerably.

She tells me the procedure will take about 40 minutes and it's very important that I don't move—at all—during that time. As part of the preparation for this procedure I'd been asked if I was claustrophobic and had said no. I've gone through this more times than I can count in the last thirty years.

As my body is moved in and out of the large machine, I do deep breathing exercises, meditate, and notice my surroundings. The ceiling has a lighted mural of the tops of trees with pink blossoms, blue sky, and fluffy white clouds. There's a loud buzzing sound, like an air conditioner. And somewhere way in the background there is music, but too faint for me to identify the song.

In the middle of the process, I have a hot flash. I'm wearing a mask because this is happening in the time of COVID. I really want to take the mask off, but I can't move. In my discomfort, I think about earlier situations in my life that may have forced me to learn to disregard outer circumstances and focus on calming my inner self.

I was three when Aunt Ruby locked me in a dark closet for hours for coloring outside the lines in my coloring book. Aunt Ruby was my mother's sister, older by eighteen months. My mother was the first of five sisters to get married and I was the first grandchild. Ruby wasn't yet married and took her jealousy of my mother out on me.

My mother had rheumatic fever as a child. This resulted in her having an enlarged heart and being limited in what she could do as an adult. She couldn't walk up a flight of stairs without resting several times. She couldn't drive and she never worked outside of the home. My mother was told she'd die if she went into labor. I was a diaphragm baby, taken out by a planned Caesarian section before labor could happen. My mother's tubes were tied so she couldn't get pregnant again.

I was named Janice, which I was told meant the grace of God. My parents believed I was a miracle sent from God to help take care of my sickly mother. From the beginning, I was told that if I upset my mother, she could die. If I spoke too loudly or had a temper tantrum, I could kill my mother. I learned to be very quiet and to be as helpful as I could be. I learned not to impose myself on others.

When I was three-years-old and my mother was in the hospital, I stayed with Aunt Ruby. I wasn't happy with this living situation, and was afraid it would be permanent if my mother died. It was during the summer and Ruby was living in a large old Victorian house that was a college dorm during the school year. We were the only two people rattling around in this cavernous building.

When I was allowed to visit my mom in the Catholic hospital, I was even more afraid for my mother's life. In her hospital room I met two of the nuns that were caring for her. They were in full habit with only their faces peeking out. I had never seen such strange creatures before. They seemed other than human and I didn't know what they were doing to my mother. I was afraid and didn't have many acceptable ways of expressing that fear.

When we got back to Ruby's living quarters after this visit, I used my coloring book to express my fears. I scribbled boldly inside and outside the lines. In Ruby's view, this was the behavior of a naughty girl who deserved punishment. Several hours locked in a pitch-black closet seemed appropriate to her.

Although I was terrified in that dark closet, I'm now grateful for the powerful early lesson that I received—*I can comfort myself.* This was one of my first experiences of creating an inner sense of calm in spite of what was happening in the world around me. I'm not at the mercy of the outside world to determine how I feel. Learning that how I feel is an inside job was empowering and has guided me through many situations (like the CT/PET scan) that could have been even more stressful.

CHAPTER TWO

Car Accident

I AM THIRTEEN-YEARS-OLD and my parents are going to drive from our home in Fresno, California, to Hillsboro, Kansas, to attend the annual Mennonite conference. Most of my father's family lives in Kansas, so this is also a chance to visit cousins I have enjoyed playing with on past family vacations. My father is adamant that I should go with them even though the trip is during the school year and I don't want to miss school. Since I'm a good student, my father insists I should skip school and join them on this trip. I work hard at being a good student, and don't want to get behind and risk losing my edge.

My father wasn't someone I could easily negotiate with. He needed to be in charge and I had learned to be an obedient daughter. When I strayed from his wishes, he didn't hesitate to spank me. I'd had two recent spankings—one for jumping on my parent's bed with some of my friends, and the other for my behavior during a Sunday morning church service. I'd been allowed to sit in the front with a girlfriend instead of with my parents, but they'd seen us whispering to each other during the service. A wooden coat hanger was the tool used to beat obedience into me.

It was unusual for me to defy or challenge my father's wishes directly, but I felt strongly enough about this trip that I refused to go. I arranged to stay with my mother's youngest sister and her husband who lived only a few blocks from us. I could still walk to my junior high school from their house.

Because I didn't go on the trip, my parents took two other passengers along—two single older adults from our church who also wanted to attend the conference in Kansas. The night they were scheduled to come home, about 9 p.m., I started crying. I said to my aunt, "Something bad has happened to my parents." This was before the days of cell phones and constant communication. She tried to reassure me that there were many possibilities that could have delayed them and she was sure they would be home tomorrow. I didn't sleep well that night.

The next morning, we were awakened at six a.m. by our minister knocking on the door. He was there to tell me that my parents had been in a serious car accident at 9 p.m. the previous evening. They were hit head-on by a driver who'd fallen asleep at the wheel. My parents were both in the hospital in the little desert town of Mojave, about 170 miles away. The two passengers were both killed in the accident. If I had been on that trip, I would have been sitting in one of the deadly seats those passengers had occupied.

The next morning my mother's cousin took me to Mojave to see my parents. My father had a deep gash in his leg from the emergency brake, but didn't have any broken bones or serious injuries. He was clearly shaken. He was in a bed in the hallway in the hospital. As he saw me approaching him, he started to cry. This was the first time I remember seeing my father cry.

I still have a vivid memory of the 1947 baby blue Plymouth that was totaled. That visual memory includes a clothes hanger that I had covered with white silk as a present for my mother. It was lying in the car, a symbol of how quickly something beautiful can be shattered.

My mother had a broken pelvis and was in a hospital bed in our home for months, while I was forced to grow up quickly. My father hardly knew how to boil water. Mom had been our cook. She often instructed me from her hospital bed as I became responsible for feeding the three of us. I didn't learn complex recipes. I mostly learned how to open cans or frozen packages and heat them on the stove. Microwaves were still something in the future.

My father's attitude towards me changed with that accident. The heated arguments we'd had before they left on that trip were replaced with trust in my judgement. He was so grateful that I wasn't in that car, and I felt a new respect from him. He was humbled and softened by that experience, and we had both gained confidence in my intuition and discernment.

CHAPTER THREE
UNDIAGNOSED ILLNESS

It is more important to know what sort of person has a disease than to know what sort of disease a person has.

~ Hippocrates

I WAS A SIXTEEN-YEAR-OLD junior in high school, loving my second year of French with a teacher who was born and raised in France, and thus fluent in French. His accent was the real thing and that was exciting because learning French from him would prepare me to one day travel in France and connect with native French speakers.

I also enjoyed my Algebra class, and quickly realized I had an aptitude for math. I was an A student who enjoyed school. I was active in the local Youth for Christ organization, went to Saturday night rallies, played my accordion at functions, and helped plan weekly morning meetings before school. Roosevelt High School was a mile from my home, close enough for me to walk to and from every day. Everything changed midyear when I started running a fever and feeling exhausted most of the time. My parents kept me home, thinking I would be better soon, but after a week with no improvement, they took me to a medical doctor. My symptoms were consistent with mononucleosis, which was common at the time. However, the doctor tested me and determined I didn't have mono. The doctor was stumped.

Medical doctors were trained to make a diagnosis in order to know what medication to use. Without a diagnosis, the doctor didn't know how to treat me, but he tried, prescribing a medicine that I think was a parasite treatment. I took several pills a day for a week, but the medicine made me vomit so much I lost about seven pounds that week. I didn't have extra pounds to lose. I was sometimes teased by the bullies at church that it took two of me to make a shadow. Besides being tired all the time, now I was feeling nauseous and weak, underweight, and still running a temperature that went up a few degrees by the end of each day. I became afraid I'd never get better.

I had missed enough school by this time, with no improvement in sight, that I was assigned a home school teacher who came to my house for a couple of hours every day. She wasn't a native French speaker, and didn't make Algebra fun. By that time, I could add depression to my list of symptoms. I felt like I was missing out in my studies, and I definitely missed seeing my friends.

Watching TV requires very little energy, so that's how I spent much of my time. Every afternoon on *The Arthur Godfrey Show*, I swooned over Pat Boone, and adored the McGuire Sisters. I lived vicariously through Annette Funicello's adventures on the *Mickey Mouse Club*. This provided the majority of my enjoyment for most of the second semester of my junior year.

Since medical doctors couldn't diagnose or help me, my parents took me to a chiropractor in Reedley, the little town where I was born, about twenty-five miles from Fresno where we lived. People joked that Reedley was the M & M town since most people living there were either Mennonites or Mexicans. Dr. Friesen had been a Mennonite missionary in South America, and he seemed old to me. He had a tiny office that smelled and looked like it hadn't changed for a long time—definitely not modern. I don't know if his assistant was a nurse, but she wore a stiff white uniform and a white nurse's hat, accentuating her stiff demeanor. She was very proper and also seemed really out of date at the time. I don't remember feeling any warmth or seeing any smiles in that office. I didn't feel hopeful about this intervention, but my parents felt hopeful because of their belief in chiropractors, who were considered alternative practitioners at that time. We had chiropractors in our family on my mother's side and I grew up hearing a story that demonstrated the value of chiropractic treatment.

As the story goes, when I was about a year old, my maternal grandparents had a car accident in Texas as they were driving from California to Oklahoma to visit relatives. My grandmother landed in the hospital with a broken back and was told she'd never walk again. Fred, her cousin in Oklahoma, who was a chiropractor, rented a hearse because he couldn't access an ambulance, drove to Texas, checked Grandma out of the hospital, and took her to his house. He put a board between the spring and mattress of a bed that she spent six weeks in as he treated her daily. She totally recovered and walked normally for the next forty years. In our family, we knew chiropractors could do miraculous things. I needed a miracle.

I felt like I was missing out on life and was desperate to be healthy again. It seemed like my best option at the time was to follow Dr. Friesen's advice that, with years of hindsight, has held up well. Dr. Friesen said *we didn't need to name my illness.* Obviously something was wrong, but our bodies are meant to heal themselves. We needed to give my body the nutrients it needed for self-healing. He rubbed minerals into my body, gave me some Chinese herbs to make a foul-tasting tea, and used a pendulum to determine what I should and shouldn't eat to strengthen my immune system.

His dietary recommendations were challenging for a sixteen-year-old, but my motivation was strong enough to persevere. I couldn't eat anything white, including sugar and white flour. No birthday cake, Twinkies, or Wonder bread, all of which I loved. (That's an indication of how bad my diet was before Dr. Friesen's intervention.) I remember going to a birthday party where carrot cake (my favorite) was served and I felt deprived as I watched everyone else enjoy it. There were also some recommendations of what to eat in addition to what I should avoid. He instructed me to eat lots of red meat, have some vinegar and nutmeg every day, and gave me a list of which vegetables were healthiest for me.

I saw Dr. Friesen weekly for several months. Each week he rubbed minerals into my body again. I don't remember how long I drank the foul-tasting tea, but I've since been exposed to Chinese medicine and recognized the concoction that Dr. Friesen prepared for me. He didn't call it Chinese herbs at the time, but I recognized the look and the smell when I visited a Chinese medicine practitioner years later.

I carefully followed Dr. Friesen's recommended diet which was a huge change from the way my mother usually cooked. Every Saturday my mother (like every good Mennonite wife) made the traditional zwieback that was part of our Mennonite culture. It was an all-day project, mixing the dough, letting it rise, making it into round buns, placing two together, one on top of the other, letting them rise again, and baking them. With the same dough she also made cinnamon rolls, rolling out the dough, sprinkling sugar and cinnamon on it, rolling it up into rolls, and smashing the rolls together in a baking pan. When it came out of the oven, she smothered the top with a powdered sugar frosting.

We didn't get to eat the cinnamon rolls until Sunday morning, but my Saturday night treat was the extra dough left over from making a pie crust. Small strips of dough were sprinkled with sugar and cinnamon and baked with the zwieback, cinnamon rolls, and pie. All of it was basically white flour and sugar—staples of our diet for many years. I felt immensely deprived when I had to give up all this comfort food. No friends, no exercise, no going out, and now no comfort food. "This better work," I thought.

After six months on this white-free diet, I was healthier than I'd ever been. My temperature was normal and I was no longer fatigued all the time. Prior to that, I used to have the flu every winter and had even had pneumonia. Following my diet change, I didn't have the flu for at least twenty years. My straight hair that my mom curled with home permanents every year was suddenly naturally curly. Life didn't just get back to normal; it got better than anything I'd ever known.

This experience had a profound and lasting impact on

me. I learned there is another way of approaching illness that doesn't depend on the pharmaceutical industry. This was my first exposure to the age-old controversy of the germ theory versus the terrain theory. The germ theory argues that germs are what we need to worry about and we need to keep finding ways to kill them off. The medical doctor I saw at sixteen needed to know what germ was attacking me before he could treat me. The terrain theory argues that if the body is well and balanced, the germs that are a natural part of life and the environment will be dealt with by the body. When an illness occurs, the body needs to be balanced and/or fortified so it can deal effectively with the germs.

This is not a new idea, but I hadn't been so personally and intimately introduced to it before. This experience stimulated my belief in the terrain theory. We never named whatever was making me sick, yet by fortifying my immune system, my symptoms were eliminated. This gave me a strong belief in the self-healing ability of my body.

I knew that my father had false teeth by the time he was thirty-years-old, and I was told that was because he ate so much sugar, but beyond the health of teeth, this was my first exposure to the idea that my overall health might be related to what I ate. This experience was a profound lesson for me that what we eat matters. For the self-healing mechanism to be effective, the body needs appropriate fuel.

When I was diagnosed with cancer many years later, the first recommendation from a doctor was to depend on the pharmaceutical industry to attack the cancer. In this case, the treatment was called chemotherapy. Of course, there is no germ that we know of that causes cancer, but the principal is the same. Attacking the cancer is similar to attacking a germ, but this ignores the terrain and the self-healing ability of the body. It destroys the very immune system that I depended on for my body to eliminate the cancer. My earlier lessons were so strong that I couldn't follow that recommendation. I did one infusion of chemotherapy out of fear, and quit when I experienced the destruction it was doing to my immune system.

Nutrition became my number one "treatment." I studied the research on nutrition and cancer, and I also worked with nutritionists that tested my body to determine what I needed. I learned that the needs of each particular body may be unique. Dr. Friesen's determination of what I needed to eat didn't come only from a book or a research study. Of course, he had knowledge from research and his years in medicine, but he also used a pendulum to personalize his suggestions to my body's needs. This lesson has come back to me over and over again in my years of living with cancer as I hear various practitioners or speakers recommend a specific diet for everyone with cancer. I know the recommendations need to be more individualized than that. My use of nutrition has evolved over the years as we have learned more. The biggest lesson may be that not everyone benefits from the same diet.

I've had phone calls and emails from many newly diagnosed cancer patients over the years. The first thing most of them want to know is what they should be eating. In 1989, when I was diagnosed, the knowledge wasn't as prevalent as it is now that what we eat affects the health of our bodies.

As I planned the programs for the *Cancer as a Turning Point, From Surviving to Thriving*™ conference, I always included a presenter on the subject of nutrition. There are some nutritional principles that all experts agree on, but that many oncologists still don't seem to be aware of. I've had an argument with an oncologist who insisted that sugar didn't affect cancer. Most doctors are not required to study nutrition and aren't experts in this field. Science is now clear that sugar feeds cancer. Most complex carbohydrates (pasta, bread, pizza) turn into sugar. There are other principles that can apply to any effort to create a healthier body. These will be discussed in another chapter.

But I didn't trust all self-proclaimed experts. I interviewed potential speakers before inviting them to participate in the conference. If they said all cancer patients needed a vegan diet, I didn't invite them to speak. If a vegan diet is the only way to health, how did my body get healthy at age sixteen when one of the big recommendations was to eat more red meat?

There is research to back up beliefs about most diets for cancer patients, and they all have anecdotes that demonstrate they're right. But if you dig deeper, there are anecdotes where any particular diet didn't work for a particular patient. In all the research, there is no diet that is healthy for 100% of the people. We each need to find out what is best for our bodies.

The lessons from my illness as a teenager were so profound that I'm grateful for the experience. There was other fallout from this experience that I wish hadn't happened, but it was worth it for the life-saving lessons I learned. When I went back to school my senior year, the native French speaking teacher was gone. My third year of French was with a teacher who couldn't speak French very well, flirted with the handsome boys in the class, and didn't pay much attention to me. Jim Hamilton, the tallest and best-looking boy in the class, got the award senior year for the best French student, although even the teacher admitted to me privately that I was a better student. When I traveled to France six years later, my French wasn't as good as it might have been if I would have had my native French speaking teacher for two years.

In a high school graduating class of 625, I just missed making it into the top ten students because during the semester I was home schooled I couldn't take a required PE course. They gave me a C for PE that semester. There was another girl in my graduating class who was blind. Because of her disability, she didn't get graded for PE and she was in the top ten. I was upset about the unfairness of this. Seemed to me that I also had a disability that semester and shouldn't be punished because of it, but the principal didn't see it my way. I was number eleven out of the class of 625. Only the top ten were publicized.

In the long run, do either of these things matter? Maybe they were gifts I can be grateful for—a great opportunity to learn to live with the unfairness that is inevitable in life. The lessons I learned through this experience about how to maintain health and support the self-healing ability of my body may have extended my life by many years.

And through the conferences I created, these lessons were passed on to thousands of others. What felt like a tragedy when I was sixteen now feels like one of the most profound experiences of my life.

I AM FIVE YEARS OLD; my friend, Patsy, and I are walking to the grocery store a few blocks from my home in the small town of Reedley where I was born. About a block from the store, on one of the busiest streets in Reedley, we witness a serious accident. A car entering the road from a driveway is broadsided by a truck going faster than it should have been.

I have a vivid memory of the dead body of a soldier, lying on the side of the road in his army uniform, with his eyeball on the ground next to him. I saw how quickly death could happen and I was scared. I wanted to be sure I would go to Heaven when my death came.

In the evangelical Christian Mennonite Brethren world I was being raised in, Heaven and Hell were certainties. Unless I accepted Jesus Christ as my personal Savior, I was on my way to Hell. I hurried home and asked my mother to pray with me as I joined the group that was assured of going to Heaven.

At age eleven, I was baptized by immersion in the local river. There were about 10 of us, all dressed in white. My parents were among other congregants witnessing the event from the shore. The minister held my nose as he lowered me into the water backwards. I officially became part of the flock, an obedient and devout member of the Mennonite Brethren Church.

There were many activities I couldn't engage in as an earnest Mennonite, including dancing, smoking, drinking, movies, card playing, and of course sex before marriage. The reason given that most of these activities were forbidden was that they were "of the devil." In retrospect, it's difficult to understand the inconsistencies. We couldn't go to movies, but we could watch TV. We couldn't dance, but we could roller skate with a partner at the skating rink. In my youth, I didn't question any of it. I followed the rules.

I went to my first movie when I was a freshman at Tabor College. Since it was a Mennonite school, going to a movie was against the rules of the college. Tabor is in Hillsboro, Kansas, and at the time there was no movie theater in Hillsboro. There were at least three Mennonite churches in Hillsboro and most people living in the small town were Mennonites.

I was part of a group of five freshman girls who drove twenty-five miles to McPherson to see "South Pacific." This was my first time in a movie theater. I was surprised to see about twenty-five other Tabor students in the theater, including some of the star basketball players. I couldn't identify what was dangerous or sinful about the movie. The music was wonderful. We bought the record and frequently played it in the student lounge. There was no rule about listening to the music, and those of us who had been at the theater gave each other knowing looks as it played.

I don't remember who got in trouble for going to the movie, but I know someone did, but the boys who played on the basketball team didn't. Our basketball team was important to the college, and the hypocrisy of letting them get by with it was the final straw that made me decide to leave Tabor College in the middle of my sophomore year. I went back to Fresno, lived with my parents, and finished college at Fresno State College with a major in psychology.

My first exposure to a more all-encompassing God was in psychology classes at Fresno State College. The head of the psychology department was a Jungian who had actually studied with Carl Jung, a contemporary of Freud. I took several classes from him, all rooted in Jungian psychology. The most interesting was Psychology of Religion. I remember watching a movie in class that included an interview with Carl Jung. The interviewer asked him if he believed in God and he replied, "No; I don't have to believe because I know that God exists." The God he knew was more loving and inclusive than the God that would allow only Christian believers into Heaven. I began questioning what I had been taught.

My senior year in college I dated Richard, who was on the way to becoming a Presbyterian minister. On July 4th, the summer after college graduation, he lied to me about why he couldn't spend the day with me. I later discovered he had spent the day with Shirley. When I confronted him about his lie, he said he'd prayed about it and God had told him not to tell me the truth. I was furious, not just because he lied to me, but because he used God as an excuse for his own inadequacy. That was the end of that relationship and another step toward questioning my Christian beliefs.

My doubts got even bigger during the next year as I

was doing a year of voluntary service for the Mennonite Central Committee. I was assigned to work at Brook Lane Psychiatric Center, a private mental hospital in Hagerstown, Maryland, run by the Mennonites. My Christian beliefs were so pervasive that I thought mental illness was the work of the devil. A belief in Jesus Christ would protect someone from mental illness.

That belief was turned upside down when I met a patient who, as a missionary in Africa, had been raping teenage girls in his congregation because "God told him to." And again, when I met a patient who had been sent home from the mission field because of her deep depression. They had both gone to the mission field because of their belief in Jesus Christ and their desire to spread that belief to others. If their faith in Jesus had protected them from mental illness, I wouldn't have met them as patients in a mental hospital.

After all those seeds of doubt had been planted, they were generously watered and fertilized when I went to graduate school at UCLA. I lived in an apartment with three other girls, one Christian and two Jewish. I learned about the apartment because of a connection with the one Christian girl, but it was the two Jewish girls who became good friends. This was my first opportunity to have deep and meaningful conversations with someone outside of my Christian tribe.

My roommate, Robbie, was shocked that I believed she was going to Hell because she was Jewish and didn't accept Jesus as her Savior. We spent hours in deep philosophical and spiritual discussions. My mind and heart were opened to a much bigger world than the one I had been steeped in during childhood. It was not easy to let go of the safety and security of the Mennonite womb. What if they were right and I was headed for eternity in hell?

As I was going through this evolution, my father (still married to my mother) had an affair with Virginia, a Mennonite woman. He denied it at first, but eventually the truth came out. He was given the opportunity to confess his sins of adultery and lying to the Board of Trustees of the church. When he refused, he was kicked out of the church. My mother got a lot of empathy and support from the church.

My mother suffered greatly and almost died, and then somehow found the strength to leave my father and move into an apartment on her own. She had never been on her own in her life. She had gone from living with her parents to marrying my father. She blossomed living alone in her apartment. After thirty years of marriage, my mother divorced my father, and he married Virginia. They were not welcome in the Mennonite church, but attended another evangelical Christian church and still claimed to be Christians.

About six months after marrying Virginia, my father, on bended knee, told my mother he had made the biggest mistake of his life and asked if she would come back to him. She replied that she loved not having anyone to answer to and had never been happier. She had no interest in being married to him again.

Virginia was the most disagreeable, unkind person I had ever met, and she claimed to be a Christian. She and my father yelled at each other constantly. When he complained to me about how mean she was and how unhappy he was, I questioned why he didn't leave. He said he wasn't about to let her have his house (that he had put her name on when they married). He asked her to leave many times, but she refused. Living in such a stressful situation, encircled by anger, I wasn't surprised that my father's health deteriorated.

When my father was in the hospital, Virginia called me to warn me that if I tried calling his doctor or getting any information about him, she would sue me. Just before my father's 80th birthday, Virginia moved him from the hospital to a nursing home, not telling me or his friends where he was. She forbade the hospital staff to tell me anything, but one of the nurses grasped the situation and told me where he was transferred. The other three members of my father's old church quartet that had sung together for decades gathered with me in his room and celebrated his birthday with him. My father couldn't speak, but as the three quartet members sang one of the songs they had sung together for years, he mouthed the words and smiled. It was a very touching moment for all of us. Virginia was furious when she found out we had visited him and cheered him up.

Virginia didn't tell me when my father died less than a year after his 80th birthday. A cousin happened to go to the nursing home to visit him a few days after his death, and my cousin contacted me with the sad news. Virginia didn't allow an obituary to be printed in the local paper. My father had been well loved by many in the community and would have had a big funeral if people knew he'd died, but Virginia allowed only a small graveside service, attended by about twenty people. Again, it was my cousin who told me about this. If it was up to Virginia, I'd have known nothing. I clung to the verse in the Bible that said, "By their fruits you shall know them. The fruits of the spirit are love, joy, peace, long suffering, gentleness, goodness and faith." I was learning that people could demonstrate those qualities no matter what their religion, and someone could claim to be a Christian without any of those qualities.

I decided I would rather spend eternity in Hell with my new loving, non-Christian friends than in Heaven with the likes of Virginia.

CHAPTER FIVE
YOU HAVE CANCER

I'M SITTING ALONE IN MY car in the parking lot of a posh surgery center in Los Gatos, California, unable to drive because I can't see through my tears. I've just heard the words, "What's going on here is serious business. You have cancer." These words have come from the mouth of a plastic surgeon, a friend of my husband, who has removed two lumps, one from my breast and one from under my arm. Both lumps had been malignant, I hadn't felt enough compassion or empathy from him to be comfortable sharing my vulnerable feelings. It wasn't until I was alone in my car that I let myself feel the impact of what he had said. I never thought I would hear those words, "You have cancer." This couldn't be happening to me. I felt afraid, alone, and devastated. It was a long time before my vision was clear enough to navigate my way home.

With my hindsight vision, I can see that my life was the perfect storm for cancer to grow. I could be a poster-child for the theory that stress is a major factor in the etiology of cancer and that it takes two or three years for it to develop. A number of events happened in 1986 that add up to a pretty traumatic year. My first cancer diagnosis was in May of 1989.

At the time of these events, I was busy dealing with

each one as it happened. In retrospect, I can see how they added up to major stress. In 1986, I lost The Center for Health Awareness, a business that I started and loved; I moved out of the first house I purchased by myself; Brian (my son) went to live with his father; we gave Chewy (our dog) away; I moved in with husband # 2 after knowing him for about six months; and we went heavily into debt starting a new business with a steep learning curve. Besides not grieving these major losses, I was also not eating a nutrient-dense diet; I wasn't exercising; I had let my social support system, my church community, and even my connection to my own soul, go by the wayside.

After terminating my seven-year career at the Center for Health Awareness, and deciding to let Brian live with his dad, I needed to figure out what to do with myself. I had started dating Michael, who was sweeping me off my feet. He was handsome, charismatic, fun, charming, and also at a crossroads in his career. Michael was just starting a temporary job in San Francisco. We had both always wanted to live in The City. Moving in together in an apartment in San Francisco seemed like the ideal solution for both of us. With my 20-20 hindsight, I can see there were red flags in that first year with Michael, indicating this might not be a healthy relationship for me. When his friend, Megan, visited us and spent the night, Michael suggested to me that we invite her to share our bed for a threesome. This didn't fit into my desires or my values, but I didn't know what a major factor that difference in values would become in our relationship. In those beginning years I didn't consider leaving Michael. Although I wasn't conscious of it at the time, the relationship with him gave me something to focus on that distracted me from the pain of my losses. My new life kept me entertained and busy enough that I could insulate myself from the pain of losing Brian and the Center for Health Awareness.

Michael and I lived in San Francisco for a year. He was consulting with Sami, the owner of a quaint and charming Bed and Breakfast on Haight Street called the Red Victorian Inn. There were some challenges happening between the owner and her staff. One morning when Michael was having a joint meeting with Sami and her staff, he asked me to come with him so I could answer the phone at the B&B during the meeting. I had fifteen minutes of training on the operations of the business after which they went into the meeting.

About an hour later, I got the news that every one of her staff had quit and I was now the person with the most experience in the business. Sami asked me if I would stay temporarily and hire new staff for her. She was not a hands-on business owner and didn't know what to do. In a way, this was a real gift for me since I had just left the Center for Health Awareness and had no income. I worked at the Red Vic part time about nine months, hiring and training staff. I learned that Sami was a challenging person to deal with, and when she asked me to stay on permanently as the manager, I said no.

In the meantime, Michael and I were planning our future. He had recently ended several years of working for NASA doing research with pilots, studying how moving through time zones affected them. This required that he travel much of the time. I had just completed seven years of traveling to teach seminars for nurses. We both wanted to stay put for a while; we wanted to work together; and we wanted to learn something new. He had a friend who owned a futon furniture store in Monterey. Futons were trendy at the time and this seemed like a business we could learn and be successful at together.

There were already too many futon stores in San Francisco, and we were discouraged by The City's cold weather. There weren't as many futon stores in San Jose and that was an area we were both familiar with. We moved into an inexpensive apartment in San Jose and opened our first California Futons store in April, 1987 in San Jose. We financed it with a second mortgage on my house (that was rented out) and maxed out our credit cards. We were open seven days a week, and it was many months before we could afford to hire any staff. Our learning curve included getting educated about our product, suppliers, merchandising, marketing, accounting, business practices, and eventually hiring and managing staff.

We were accomplishing our goal of working together and learning something new. It seemed like we were passionate about our business, but in retrospect, I'd say we were driven. For the first couple of years, I forgot everything I knew about nurturing myself. I worked seven days a week, ten to twelve hours a day. I didn't go to concerts, picnics, movies, leisurely dinners, or vacations. Not even a walk on the beach or hike in the mountains. I didn't attend the funeral of an ex-employee because I thought I couldn't afford to take time away from the business. I had been an avid reader, but I don't think I read a single book during this time. Life was about California Futons.

Our store was surrounded by fast food outlets and that's where most of my meals came from. Dairy Queen next door, McDonalds across the street, and Wendy's a block away. And on the way home to our apartment a few blocks away, there was Kentucky Fried Chicken and A&W Root Beer. I didn't have time or energy to shop or cook healthy meals.

When I felt a lump in my left breast, I had a mammogram. My doctor called me to say she didn't think it was cancer and no need to do anything about it. She called me at home the night before she was leaving on a trip to France. I think she may have been preoccupied. If I knew then what I know now, I would have had it biopsied then, but I wanted so much for it to be nothing that I believed her. I didn't give it another thought and went on living my stressful life.

About six months later when I also felt a lump under my left arm, I knew it wasn't a good sign. I asked my friend Anna who was a nurse to feel the lumps, and she was adamant that I needed to get both lumps biopsied. I didn't have much money, and I didn't have health insurance.

Michael had a friend who was a plastic surgeon with his own operating suite, and Michael arranged a good deal to remove and biopsy both lumps. When the three of us were together in the surgeon's swank office, making the plans, most of the conversation was about airplanes and flying stories since that was the connection the two men had. I felt like what was going on with my body was of little interest, and certainly couldn't be serious. We were just making a business deal.

I was so out of touch with my feelings that I didn't consider taking anyone with me to my appointment to get the results of the biopsies. I couldn't ask Michael to go with me since someone had to run the store. California Futons still seemed more important than my body. Because my life was so consumed with working in the business, I hadn't put my time or energy into nourishing or even maintaining my friendships. Even if I did think of taking someone with me, there was no one else in my life at the time that I felt comfortable in asking to accompany me to the appointment.

The surgeon referred me to an oncologist who I saw the next week. Looking very professional in his white coat, and speaking in a German accent, he recommended a mastectomy and chemotherapy, starting immediately. I asked him for an estimate of what the total course of treatment would cost and he estimated $10,000. I had no health insurance and little money, and a strong belief in the self-healing ability of the body. I looked for books that would give me clues as to how others had dealt with similar situations, but there wasn't much available in 1989.

I needed to decide what to do about this new uninvited guest in my body. At the time I felt like my body had betrayed me. In retrospect, I think I had betrayed my body.

CHAPTER SIX

CANCER TREATMENTS

My INITIAL BREAST CANCER DIAGNOSIS was in May, 1989. Michael and I had a Hawaiian trip planned for June. Friends of his had invited us to stay with them in their "cottage" (turned out to be a big house) on Hanalei Bay in Kauai. This would be our first vacation since starting our retail furniture business two years earlier that kept us working seven days a week. We had employees who could run the business and we were finally going to get away. But I had a serious dilemma—I wasn't willing to give up this trip, and I wasn't willing to be on the beach in Kauai with a disfigured body.

Since I wasn't willing to have the mastectomy immediately, the oncologist recommended I start chemotherapy right away and have a mastectomy when I returned from my Hawaiian vacation. This doctor made it clear he thought there was an urgency to start treatment, immediately. I was resistant to having chemotherapy because of my belief in the self-healing mechanism of the body, but I was also afraid of the cancer. I felt like I had to do something and I didn't know what else to do. My fear made the decision and I started chemo.

After only one infusion and a week of daily pills, I had mouth sores and my hair started coming out in clumps. I knew this was compromising my immune system, the very self-healing strategy that I most needed now. I remembered what I had learned at age sixteen about the self-healing mechanisms of the body—my body knows how to heal itself and needs the fuel and care to create a terrain not conducive to the growth of cancer.

When I asked my oncologist for statistics on the effectiveness of this chemo, he said it would increase my chances of survival by five percent. I decided it wasn't worth it to destroy my immune system for such a small potential benefit, so I went on that Hawaii trip knowing that I wouldn't continue chemotherapy when I returned.

My hair continued to come out in clumps during the vacation. When I was visiting a lighthouse, standing on a windy outcropping of land, clumps of my hair blew out to sea. I needed a wig by the end of that trip, but waited until I got home to buy one. I only wore it a couple of days in the California heat and decided my comfort eclipsed how I looked. I had my hair cut really short and was grateful it didn't *all* come out.

The other medical recommendation was to have a mastectomy. In my thirties, I had done some traveling with Barbara, who had had a radical mastectomy years before we met. We shared hotel rooms and hot tubs, and I got a good look at the long-term consequences of her cancer treatment. Her chest caved in where she used to have a breast and her entire right arm was twice as big as her other one. Her disfigured body distressed me.

When I heard the surgeon say, "You have cancer," Barbara's scar was one of my first images. My initial reaction to having breast cancer wasn't a fear of death; it was a fear of being disfigured. I hadn't known anyone who had died from breast cancer, but I was familiar with how a body looked following a mastectomy.

After being diagnosed in May, doing one round of chemo in early June, and enjoying our Hawaiian vacation, I was still feeling resistant to further treatment. My strong belief in the self-healing ability of the body made me wonder if I could make the cancer disappear by employing psycho-spiritual techniques. In July I attended a workshop at the Palace of Fine Arts in San Francisco with Brugh Joy, one of my New Age gurus. I had read his book, *Joy's Way*, and knew he focused on the whole self—mind, body, and spirit. If there was a way to heal this cancer using spiritual methods, he would lead me in that direction.

When he asked the audience who would like to come up on the stage and work with him as a demonstration, about fifty out of 900 people raised their hands. He asked the fifty of us to put our names in a basket and he would pull one out to work with. I had a premonition that he would pick me, and he did. It was a dream come true to be able to talk one on one with Brugh Joy about my cancer and my life. I didn't care that there were 900 people listening. I thought this would point me in the direction of healing at the psychological, spiritual level, where I believed true healing happened.

After our conversation, he invited people from the audience to join us on stage; hundreds of people surrounded me and did a "healing ceremony." Other people remarked on the great energy they felt, *but I didn't feel anything*. What stands out to me about that experience was his statement to me in private after the healing ceremony. He said what I was dealing with was big. He recommended that I have a mastectomy. That message, coming from him, was what I needed to move forward.

Since I didn't have health insurance at the time, I had to rely on the kindness of friends. My husband had a friend who was an anesthesiologist at a local hospital. He didn't charge me for his services. He recruited a surgeon friend of his who charged me half price. I had a mastectomy in August, but not the radical version Barbara had suffered. By this time, they had learned to do modified radical mastectomies so they didn't cut the muscles. Because I didn't have health insurance, I needed the least expensive surgery and that couldn't include reconstruction. I had a mastectomy as an outpatient (23 hours in the hospital) for a total cost of $2,000 and went home flat chested on my left side.

At that time, most women stayed in the hospital about three days for a mastectomy. Since I was going home earlier, I thought I might need some help when I got home. Michael would be going to work at the furniture store twelve hours a day and I would be home alone. I hired someone to come help me, and then felt the stress of trying to figure out what she should do. I really didn't need help. I let her go after only one day.

My biggest discomfort came not from the mastectomy, but from having twelve lymph nodes removed under my arm to determine if the cancer had spread. I had a drain that had to be emptied periodically; when it was full, it felt like I had a bowling ball under my arm. My range of motion was limited and I couldn't drive for two weeks. My doctor gave me exercises to do to increase my range of motion and prescribed pain pills. He said, "Take the pain pills for two weeks whether you think you need them or not. If you don't take them, the exercises will cause pain and you won't do them, leaving you with permanent range of motion limitations."

I took the pain pills and spent time each day crawling my fingers up the wall as high as I could go, expanding my reach daily. By the end of two weeks, I had full range of motion.

During those first few weeks, I was in my bedroom having a conversation with my thirteen-year-old son, Brian. He was in the middle of telling me a story when I needed to change clothes. I went into my walk-in closet thinking I could change in private and still hear him. He followed me in and kept talking. He had grown up with a hot tub at home and summer vacations in the hot tubs of Tassajara Hot Springs, so nudity had been comfortable for us.

I told him if he stayed in there he would see my "ugly." He stayed. I took off my top, revealing my scar that I thought was ugly. He glanced at it, said "that's not so bad," and continued his story. That moment was immensely healing for me.

When I declined to continue with chemotherapy, the very authoritarian and aloof German oncologist gave me a prescription for Tamoxifen, standard treatment for estrogen-receptive positive breast cancer. Medication was the only tool he had been given in medical school and I couldn't believe in it.

I still craved information on how I could stimulate the self-healing ability of my body. What I also may have needed at that time was some empathy and a conversation of the heart, but that didn't seem to be in my doctor's toolbox either. I longed for a practitioner who could meet me at all levels of body, mind, and spirit. It would be a few years before I found such a person. In the meantime, I felt like I was on my own.

From my earlier experience with my undiagnosed illness, I knew that what I put in my mouth mattered. I found a nutritionist that specialized in working with cancer patients and I started paying closer attention to my diet. She recommended a vegetarian, low-fat diet, which at that time was recommended for anyone with breast cancer. I started cooking more at home, and reading labels on packaged food to be sure less than thirty percent of my calories came from fat. Knowing what I know now, that wasn't a healthy diet for me. But it was probably better than surviving on fast foods. It didn't change my terrain enough to keep the cancer from continuing to grow.

A year later I felt another lump under the same arm. A biopsy revealed that it was cancer. Since it was a local recurrence, and not systemic, the recommendation was radiation. By this time, I had health insurance. I couldn't get health insurance as an individual because of my pre-existing cancer, but we now had employees in our furniture store. By getting health insurance for the whole company, they didn't look at pre-existing conditions or require individual exams. I was covered.

The local Kaiser in Fresno didn't have a radiation

department at the time, so they paid for me to have radiation in another local health system. I had radiation on my left chest every weekday for seven weeks. In the beginning I left my orange Saab Sonnet (sports car no longer made) with the valet who parked it and then retrieved it for me after my appointment. It didn't take very many days for him to notice that my appointments were only fifteen minutes long and it wasn't worth his time to move my car to the parking garage. He started blocking off a parking space right in front of the door with an orange cone. As he saw me driving up at the same time every morning, he removed the cone with a big smile and welcomed me to my radiation treatment. His warmth and care made me feel so special that I actually looked forward to arriving at the hospital each morning. A part of me was disappointed when radiation ended and I didn't get to feel like a queen every morning.

As I started experiencing the pain of a burned chest, one of the radiation nurses gave me a tube of Aloe Vera cream she had received as a sample. She didn't know if it worked, but I could try it. Her kindness touched my heart and the Aloe Vera reduced my inflammation, but I still couldn't tolerate wearing a bra. I wore loose shirts so nothing would be painfully tight on my chest, and no one could tell I was flat chested on one side. I also exploited the power of distraction. Wearing tight pants drew attention to my lower anatomy and my unbalanced chest wasn't the center of attention.

After the radiation was finished, I got my first oncologist with my new Kaiser insurance. An older man, he was the only oncologist in the Fresno Kaiser system. When I had my mastectomy a year before this, I would have chosen to also have reconstruction if I had health insurance that would pay for it. Since I didn't, I asked my new doctor about the possibility of having reconstruction now. I was shocked by his response. *He said if I wanted both sides to look the same, I should have the other breast cut off and I could stuff Kleenex in my bra.* I couldn't believe what I was hearing. I was furious. I wrote a letter of complaint to Kaiser Customer Service. To their credit, I never had to see that doctor again. Kaiser paid for me to see another oncologist in the community who was much more knowledgeable and compassionate. His response to the same question was that reconstruction was no longer possible because I'd had radiation and that made it impossible to connect the blood vessels to create a reconstructed breast.

Of course, I was disappointed, but by this time I had spent more than a year looking at my new body and was accustomed to being flat on one side. As the years progressed, my scar and I definitely learned to live together. I used to go to Tassajara Hot Springs every summer and soak in the healing waters. I started putting temporary tattoos where I used to have a breast to let people know it was okay to look. I no longer thought of it as ugly.

After dinner at Tassajara, the men's baths were co-ed so I joined my husband and had conversations with other people in and around the tub. The day after one of those hot tub conversations, at a group meal, the subject of my mastectomy came up. A man I had conversed with the night before in the tub said he hadn't noticed that I was one-breasted. What a surprise, and how comforting to know I didn't have to lead with my scar. It didn't define me.

After the radiation, it was four years before I felt another lump under my arm, and then the lumps appeared every year or two for about eight years. Each time I had an outpatient surgery to remove the lump. Each time the biopsy revealed it was a local recurrence of cancer. During this time, I hadn't yet realized that for me cancer was a chronic illness and wasn't going away. Each recurrence instigated the same emotions as if it was a new cancer. "Oh, shit. Not again." The cancer seemed relentless and I was emotionally exhausted. Thankfully, my curiosity was always active and I continually asked what else I could do to activate the self-healing mechanism of my body.

My oncologist offered the tools he had been trained in. The cancer was estrogen receptor positive breast cancer, meaning that my cancer fed on estrogen. In order to reduce my estrogen, he recommended Tamoxifen. When this had been offered to me a year earlier, I'd said no. This time, after experiencing a recurrence of cancer, I felt even more afraid. I took Tamoxifen for five years, followed by Arimidex for three years—both medications that are designed to reduce estrogen.

During this time, I found the doctor I had been looking for from the beginning. My friend, Anna, told me about a doctor one of her friends had just married. Dwight McKee, MD, had been active as a family doctor for twelve years, learning and using alternative medicine. Now he was in the process of getting double board-certified in hematology and oncology. I first saw him at Scripps in San Diego where he was doing a residency and I was excited and relieved to discover he had abundant tools in his toolbox. He was an empathetic, caring person who understood that I was a whole person, not just a body. Our appointment ended with a heartfelt hug and I felt like I finally had someone on my team that added real value.

When Dr. McKee finished his residency, he moved to Montana. This was before the days of telemedicine, so he found creative ways of treating cancer patients around the country. He worked with and through other doctors. I was living in Santa Cruz by this time so he treated me through Randy Baker, MD, a local doctor. I saw Dr. Baker in Santa Cruz who consulted with Dr. McKee on a regular basis. Dr. McKee ordered blood tests and prescribed and monitored my treatment.

Dr. Baker's office was a couple of blocks from where I lived. I had passed it many times before going there as a patient, but didn't know it was a doctor's office. It was a modest, unassuming blue house on a corner. When I first approached the front door, I was surprised by a sign that instructed me not to enter if I had any fragrance on my body. The sign said any fragrance could make their chemically sensitive patients sick. I had a friend with chemical sensitivities that prevented her from going most places and I knew how challenging it was for her to find doctors that acknowledged her illness as real. That sign told me that Dr. Baker would be an unusual doctor.

His office was unconventional, as was he. He had long hair, always wore Birkenstocks, and his office was covered with piles of books and papers. Often when I asked a question, he would say he had just read a research study that answered that. He would go to one of maybe twelve stacks of books and papers, reach somewhere into the middle, and take out the study and read it to me. Those piles were more effective than some people's filing systems! He knew what was in there and exactly where it was. I always learned something each time I met with him.

We experimented with a number of cutting-edge treatments. Some people would call them alternative. Some people would call them illegal since in California it is only legal to treat cancer with surgery, chemotherapy, or radiation. I call them open minded, evidence-based, and potentially life-saving. For a year I had a daily injection of interferon or interleukin directly into the space under my arm where the lumps kept appearing. Dr. McKee thought there might be a sanctuary in there that my immune system couldn't get to. My husband gave me the daily injections. They were painful, but at the same time created an opportunity for an intimate experience with Michael.

For several months I drank a foul-tasting intense soy drink that came from Germany. Dr. McKee was always reading the latest research, and he spent time in Europe learning what new treatments were being discovered. I know I took lots of supplements during this time, but don't remember all their names.

During those eight years of playing whack-a-mole with removing repeated under-arm cancerous lumps, eating a vegetarian low-fat diet, taking estrogen blockers, and trying various alternative treatments, I don't know what, if anything, made a difference. It's possible I just have a slow growing cancer and it would have grown just as slowly if I had done nothing. I'd like to believe that all my efforts were beneficial, but I'll never know. That's part of the mystery of living with cancer as a chronically-recurring illness. We work as diligently as we can to discover and evaluate the various treatment options available to us and choose the ones that feel right for us without ever really knowing which ones work.

It wasn't until 2002 when I had another local recurrence in addition to a new cancer in the other breast that I altered my strategy. First, I had to deal with the lump that turned out to be a new cancer in the other breast. By that time research indicated that there was no difference in long-term outcome if I had a mastectomy or a lumpectomy. My decision to have a lumpectomy wasn't based on wanting to save my breast because of how I looked, but because of how I felt. My nipple is a cherished part of my sexual experience. It was important to me to save it.

That surgery was also a valuable lesson in how important it is to be informed and to be one's own advocate. I loved the surgeon who had taken out my annual underarm lumps. Since she had just retired, I was referred to a new surgeon. He informed me that he would take out many lymph nodes under my arm along with the lumpectomy. That had been done on the other side with my mastectomy in 1989 and I was still having an issue with lymphedema. I didn't want to repeat those challenges on the right side. I had learned about a new procedure called a sentinel node biopsy in which they determine which lymph node the cancer would go to first if it traveled, and remove only that one. I asked him to do that instead.

He argued with me, saying he didn't think I would have lymphedema, and insisted on taking out many lymph nodes to determine if the cancer had spread. I requested another surgeon who would do what I wanted. He finally admitted he didn't know how to do a sentinel node biopsy, referred me to a surgeon who did, and asked me if he could be in the surgery so he could learn. I said he could be in the room to observe as long as he didn't participate in the surgery.

The pathology reports from both the lumpectomy and sentinel node biopsy revealed cancer. That's when I altered my strategy again and changed almost everything in my life. I left my marriage, quit working at the furniture store, moved from Santa Cruz to Sacramento, made Healing Journeys (the non-profit that supported the *Cancer as a Turning Point Conference*™) my full-time job, engaged with a spiritual community, and radically changed my diet (see Nutrition chapter).

With these changes as my treatment, it was again four years before I had another local recurrence on the right side. I have not had another local recurrence on the left side since 2002. It seems these changes in my life were at least as effective as radiation in giving me four years without cancer progression.

CHAPTER SEVEN

CANCER AS A DISEASE OF THE SOUL

We are spiritual beings on a human path rather than human beings who
may or may not be on a spiritual path.

~ Teilhard de Chardin

I'M SITTING IN AN AUDITORIUM at the Disneyland Hotel in Southern California with 900 other health professionals—doctors, nurses, and social workers. Jean Shinoda Bolen, MD, a Jungian analyst and prolific author, is speaking. She's using mythology as a metaphor for illness and she says all illnesses are diseases of the soul. She's the first person I hear use the Teilhard de Chardin quote above. I feel like she's talking directly to me as my tears flow throughout her talk. At the end, I'm amazed by the standing ovation from all 900 health professionals. Clearly, her message is resonating with everyone.

I'm at this conference for continuing education as a social worker, but I'm also a cancer patient. When I was diagnosed with breast cancer in 1989, I knew there was more to healing than surgery, radiation, and chemotherapy. I'd come from a background of teaching mind/body health concepts to nurses through the Center for Health Awareness. Now a cancer patient, I was searching for strategies and support in healing my whole self—mind, body, soul, and spirit.

I had told my Kaiser oncologist that the only treatments he was recommending were focused on the body. When I asked how he was going to treat the rest of me, he raised his voice and yelled, "Emotions have nothing to do with this!" I was shocked at that response. I knew it wasn't true, but what about all the women who may hear this message and believe it? I was concerned for them. I know men get breast cancer too, but at the time my concern was women. The seed was planted during that Disneyland conference for me to create a similar event, but for those of us on the front lines dealing with cancer instead of for health professionals only.

Putting together my needs as a cancer patient with my background of teaching workshops for the Center for Health Awareness, I created a conference addressing the whole person. We had taught a seminar at the Center called "The Turning Point." I wanted to call this new program *Cancer as a Turning Point, From Surviving to Thriving*™.

During the time that my plans were being formulated, I was walking on a beach in Maui when I saw someone reading a book entitled *Cancer as a Turning Point*, by Lawrence LeShan, PhD. I thought, "Oh, shit, someone has used my title." Of course, I got the book, read it, and loved it. This was exactly the information I had been looking for, about healing beyond the limitations of medical treatments. I knew I would have to get Dr. LeShan's permission to use that title, but more about that later.

In *Cancer as a Turning Point*, Dr. LeShan wrote about the results of his fifty years of mind-body cancer research. He was a psychotherapist who wanted to determine if psychotherapy would make a difference in the progression of cancer. He was allowed to work only with patients who had been determined to be terminal. His peers said if ther-

apy might be strong enough to make a differ[ence]
possibly also be a negative difference. But, if [...]
already terminal, it didn't matter.

In the beginning of his research, he did traditional
psychodynamic psychotherapy as originated by Freud. Although Dr. LeShan's patients may have died more at peace,
they still all died as predicted. Then he decided to try a new
kind of therapy. Instead of dealing with past traumas, he focused on the patients' dreams and what would make them
excited to get up in the morning. His basic message to the
patients was, "Don't worry about what the world wants of
you. Worry about what makes you come alive because what
the world needs is people who are more alive."

When he changed the focus of therapy, 50 percent of
his terminal patients went into long-term remission. His
book is full of stories of these patients, and I was inspired.
Some of them made big changes in their lives, like changing jobs or leaving a husband. Others made small changes,
like finally taking up playing the piano which had been a
life-long dream.

Dr. LeShan said, "It is essential that the person first
learns to sing their own song fully and then, as part of their
human needs, finds a way to express their spiritual concern
with others or with the human race as a whole. Only in this
way do we act and live as a coherent whole and only in this
way can we strengthen and mobilize our self-healing and
self-repair abilities."

Reading *Cancer as a Turning Point* reinforced my belief
that there was more to healing than chemotherapy, surgery,
and radiation. I asked myself what changes I could make in

my life that would allow me to feel more alive. I knew the job I was doing—owning and managing a furniture store with my husband—was not singing my own song. I was trying to harmonize with my husband by working in the business that was his dream, not mine.

By watering and nurturing the seed that had been planted at the Disneyland conference, I discovered my own song. I formed a non-profit, Healing Journeys, and produced the first *Cancer as a Turning Point, From Surviving to Thriving*™ conference in 1994 in Monterey, California. This work became a huge part of my own healing, provided me with meaning and purpose in life, and generated more social support than I could have imagined.

Early Stepping Stones

CHAPTER EIGHT

MATH MAJOR TO MSW

MRS. MUNSON, MY MATH TEACHER in the 8th grade, was as round as she was tall, and she was not user-friendly. After a year in her class, I thought I was really stupid at math. In the 9th grade, instead of taking algebra like the college-bound kids did, I took remedial math. The teacher was relaxed, didn't expect much from us, and it was easy for me. It didn't occur to me that I might be good at math.

Then I went to high school for the 10th grade and was required to take algebra if I wanted to go to college. Surprisingly, it was not only fun, but was also pretty easy for me. It was so fun that I decided to take geometry in my junior year. My teacher, Mr. Gaither, was a tall, wiry redhead who made geometry fun. He is by far my favorite teacher of all time. When the unruly boys in the class were noisy, instead of raising his voice, Mr. Gaither whispered. It wasn't long until everyone else was quiet. He had cleverly tricked them into wanting to hear what he was saying.

By the time I started college, I was a math major, excelling in trigonometry and calculus. My freshman year in Tabor College I got the math award for the best math student in the department, in spite of being the only female.

This was not necessarily a desirable thing for me, though. I had a crush on a boy in my calculus class and occasionally approached him in the library to ask for help with our calculus homework. I'd usually find myself explaining calculus to him! I quickly learned that most boys aren't attracted to girls who appear to be smarter than they are.

By the middle of my sophomore year in college, I was bored with math and fascinated with psychology. I graduated with a major in Psychology and a minor in Math. My college professors encouraged me to go to graduate school in psychology research, saying my math background made me a perfect candidate to go into research. But that didn't interest me any more than Math did.

I knew a BA degree in Psychology wasn't enough for a career, and graduate school would be required, but I didn't know what career would be fulfilling for me. I didn't even know what the options were. I was still a Mennonite at the time. The Mennonite Central Committee did work all over the world and I applied to be a volunteer for a year, hoping they would send me to some exotic far-away country. I was ready for some adventure in my life before starting the next leg of my academic trajectory.

A foreign assignment would have been exciting, but the assignment I got turned out to help guide me towards a meaningful career. My year of voluntary service for the Mennonite Central Committee was working in a private psychiatric hospital in Hagerstown, Maryland. That was far enough away from California to be an adventure. Traveling from California to Baltimore, Maryland, was my first time in an airplane.

I lived in the nurses' quarters at the hospital for that

year. The hospital campus was in a beautiful rural setting. My walk to work was about the distance of a city block, but it was a path along the creek, with more pronounced seasonal changes than I had ever witnessed in California. For the first six months, I had a roommate from Sweden who was excited to spend six months in the United States, a foreign adventure for her. The second six months I had a roommate from the Netherlands. Having these foreign roommates allowed me to experience the customs and people from Sweden and the Netherlands without having to leave the country, but this only increased my desire for travel. I wanted to visit both of these women in their native countries.

Working as a psychiatric aide in the hospital, I got to experience what the different professions actually did in their day-to-day jobs. I observed the psychiatrist, psychologist, nurses, chaplain, and social worker. The social worker's job by far seemed the most interesting and beneficial. When I wanted to talk to a therapist that year, it was the social worker I sought out.

The social worker didn't see the patient as an individual unit, but as part of a family system. He said if you treat the patient in isolation and send her back to the family without any family intervention, the same situation is likely to evolve again. He tried to bring the family in as part of treatment. This approach made the most sense to me, and I felt excited about learning how to do that.

I applied for Social Work graduate school at UCLA. I not only was accepted, I got a scholarship. It was only $200 a month, but in 1965, that was enough to live on. I shared a house with three other female students, close enough to campus that I didn't need a car.

My second year at UCLA, I had a stipend from the state of California for $300 a month. I was told there would be some delay in starting to receive this money, so I took out a $500 interest-free loan to tide me over. Then the stipend kicked in sooner than expected. Instead of returning the $500, I used it to travel in Europe for three months before starting my second year. At that time, using the guide to Europe for $5 a day, it was possible to do this.

I visited Rigmor (my Swedish roommate) in her small hometown. I was greeted warmly by her parents who didn't speak English, and her shy younger sister who had studied English but was afraid to practice it with an American. Some of their family friends came to their home to greet me and bring me presents. They had never seen an American before. What a treat to be shown around by people who called Sweden home.

I'm grateful that my roommate from the Netherlands (Emma) traveled with me in Europe for one month. Her fluency in German came in handy when I got sick in Vienna and needed to go to a German speaking doctor. He said I had the German measles! All I saw of Vienna was the inside of my hotel room.

After the month of traveling together, I visited Emma in the orphanage where she worked. When I had lunch with the children, Emma gave me a lesson on Dutch customs. She warned me not to eat my bread with my hands because the children would laugh at me, thinking I didn't know my manners. I needed to cut my bread with a fork and knife, and put it in my mouth with my fork. From the children's perspective, I was demonstrating good manners.

My fluency in math came in handy during the second year of graduate school. A course in Statistics was required and I think I was the only person in the program who didn't have trouble with that course.

The stipend I received from the State of California came with the requirement that I would work for the State for at least a year after graduation. That first job after receiving my Masters in Social Work was for Agnews State Hospital in San Jose, California. I was on my way to a fulfilling and exciting career as a Psychiatric Social Worker and therapist.

~

CHAPTER NINE

EXPRESSION

WHEN I WAS TWO OR three years old, my mom gave me five pennies at the beginning of the week with the threat of taking a penny away any time I had a temper tantrum. She was so proud of what a fast learner I was. She had to take only one penny away and I never had another temper tantrum. I had a motivation even greater than wanting to keep the pennies, but I'm sure the money facilitated my quick learning. As a child I was told that if I did or said something that upset my mother, she could die. She'd had rheumatic fever as a child, and that had left her with an enlarged and weak heart, a leaky valve, and a tenuous hold on life. She didn't drive, didn't work outside of the home, and couldn't walk up a flight of stairs without resting several times. She said I was a gift from God to help her in her life. It was a huge responsibility for a child, and also set me up to believe that God sent me here for a purpose. I felt special, and responsible to use that specialness to benefit others.

This also set me up not to express myself. Learning not to express my negative feelings carried over to not expressing *any* feelings. Or even any opinions. I've always been described as quiet, and for good reason. I didn't want to risk killing my mother, or anybody else. The safest course of action was not to impose myself on anyone in any way.

Stay under the radar. I was told that, as a child, I used to hide under the table when visitors came to our house. My third-grade teacher told my parents that she didn't realize I was smart until halfway through the school year because I never spoke up.

My parents complained that when I unwrapped a Christmas present, they couldn't tell if I liked it or not. When I was six, I really wanted red galoshes so I could tromp through water puddles on my way to school. When I opened them on Christmas morning, I loved them, but my parents had no way of knowing that. My training not to express myself overruled a little kid's natural exuberance at getting a special Christmas present.

After not expressing myself throughout childhood, when I got to college where a public speaking class was required for graduation, I was terrified. Just thinking about getting in front of a group of people and speaking left me with a churning stomach. I put it off until the last semester. Our first assignment was a brief autobiography. Since we went in alphabetical order, I was first. I had diarrhea the night before and dreaded going to school that day. I was shaking when I got in front of the class.

My fear was a good motivator. Because of my fear, I was super prepared. I had written a good five-minute talk and had my note cards ready to prompt me in case I forgot what I was saying. I started out by saying I was born the day after Pearl Harbor. To my surprise, almost everyone else started their presentations by saying how long after Pearl Harbor they were born. I hadn't purposively imposed myself, but clearly, I had an impact on the people in the class.

Having such an effect on everyone's talks left me feeling both uncomfortable and powerful. I got an A in the class. I was less afraid of public speaking after this, but not comfortable enough that I would have chosen a career that involved speaking in front of a thousand or more people on a regular basis. Unexpectedly, such a career chose me.

I frequently prayed the Prayer of St. Francis, "Lord, make me an instrument." And always added, *show me what to do to use my gifts and talents in a way that benefits humanity*. Ironically, my cancer diagnosis may have been an answer to that prayer. My diagnosis led me to crave information, hope, support, and inspiration. I knew first-hand what a cancer patient needed. I couldn't find what I needed in the cancer world, and when I found it elsewhere, I was compelled to bring it to the cancer world. The *Cancer as a Turning Point, From Surviving to Thriving*™ conference was born as a result of my need.

I still didn't see myself as a speaker at the conferences, but I was the emcee and the conference weaver, setting the tone for the conference, and introducing the presenters. I was always nervous before going on stage, but once I got there, I had a job to do. I was focused on what the audience needed, and why I was there.

If I'd have seen a job description for what I was doing, I'd have thought I wasn't qualified and wouldn't have applied for the job. The conference started out small; I didn't know it would evolve to audiences of over a thousand. Since the conference was born from my seeing a need and filling it, I felt so guided that I never questioned whether I could do the job. This felt like my assignment from a Higher Source.

For twenty-five years, producing the *Cancer as a Turning Point*™ conference gave me a strong purpose for living. I was confident that I was fulfilling my goal of being an instrument. I felt supported and guided by a Force greater than me. I can't imagine a more rewarding career.

Our final *Cancer as a Turning Point*™ conference was in 2018. For the first time, I invited someone else to be the emcee and conference weaver, and I became a speaker. The theme of that last conference was healing stories. I had finally been convinced that my story was inspiring and educational, even though I wasn't cancer-free. I had come to believe that my story about thriving while living with cancer for over thirty years is a story worth telling. A standing ovation confirmed that.

Even as I write this memoir, the feedback I get from my writing group is that I need to be more expressive. They want more of me. I'm an old hand at not expressing feelings, and habits are hard to change.

CHAPTER TEN

PACKING PEACHES

IT WAS THE SUMMER AFTER high school graduation and I was college bound. It was assumed I would go to one of the two Mennonite colleges—Pacific College in Fresno, where we lived, or Tabor College in Hillsboro, Kansas. I didn't consider any other option. If I went to Pacific College, I could live with my parents and save a lot of money. This is what my parents wanted me to do.

At the time, my desire to go to college was partially motivated by my longing to leave my father's house. I saw my father as shallow, prejudiced, demanding respect that I felt he hadn't earned, and not someone I would choose to live with. I dreamed of not being under his roof and in his control anymore. Tabor College seemed like the perfect solution. I had some favorite cousins living in Kansas that we had visited frequently as a child, so going that far away from home didn't feel at all scary.

My parents agreed to send me money every month for incidentals, but I had to pay for college tuition and the dorm myself. That meant I needed a job. After high school graduation, because I didn't immediately start job hunting, my father pushed me, saying I wasn't going to get a job hanging around home. But he was wrong. Within a week of "hanging around at home," I got a phone call from Walter, a man at church who was putting together a crew to pack peaches for the summer. Was I interested? Walter's phone call felt like another example of the Divine Guidance I've experienced so many times in my life.

That started a career of two summers of packing peaches. That first summer there were four of us on the crew. The other three were girls I knew from church and we had a lot of fun together. We stood on a trailer, two on one side and two on the other. The trailer had a roof on it to protect us from the beating sun and it was pulled by a tractor through the peach orchard. The Mexican pickers dumped their buckets of peaches into huge boxes in between the two sides of the trailer. We arranged the peaches in different boxes according to size. When a box was full, we stacked it up ready to ship out. We were paid by the piece. The faster we moved, the more money we made.

It could easily be over 100 degrees in Fresno in the summer and of course, there was no air conditioning in the peach orchard! Our sweaty bodies attracted peach fuzz like Velcro. This was physically miserable, but emotionally energizing. We made it fun. We covered our bodies with baby powder to keep the peach fuzz at bay, and sometimes when we encountered a hose, we had great water fights. All these years later, I still can't eat a peach with the skin on. The touch of the fuzz on my mouth makes me feel like I'm back in that peach orchard, itching all over.

Mary Ellen, one of the other crew members, was going to be my roommate at Tabor College. We were motivated to make this both profitable and fun. There's a song we used to sing at church that started, "It will be worth it all when we see Jesus." We changed the words to "It will be worth it all when we see Tabor." We sang and laughed our way through three months of fuzzy heat, and it was worth it all. We both saw Tabor College in September.

CHAPTER ELEVEN

CORKY

I AM ENJOYING WATCHING THE Chinese New Year's parade from a second story window in a hotel on the parade route in San Francisco. I'm with about fifteen other people, friends of the boyfriend who reserved the room for this occasion. Corky the clown is with me. Corky is about 10 inches tall, looking very cute with his bright yellow and orange clown outfit, red nose, and happy smile, sucking his thumb.

It's not unusual to have Corky with me. He's been traveling everywhere with me since I got him at a conference about the healing power of laughter and play, on the Queen Mary in Long Beach, California. One of the opening speakers, Carl Simonton, asked the audience what we had brought with us to play with. We had all traveled a distance from home, and what was going to amuse us on this trip? I had nothing with me to play with, so I made a trip to the hotel gift store. Corky was the perfect solution. He reminded me to have a playful attitude.

Months later, at the San Francisco hotel, Corky was passed around during the parade, and many people admired and coveted him. He was really cute. After the parade, the boyfriend who hosted the party and I were the last ones to leave. As we were gathering our belongings, Corky wasn't to be found. Someone else in that group must have decided Corky should go home with them. I didn't know most of these people and had to surrender to never seeing Corky again. I was heartbroken.

I looked at several stores for another Corky and couldn't find one. Corky had a tag on him and I remembered the name of the company that made him, so I contacted them. I could get one wholesale from the company if I ordered a box of twenty, in a variety of colors.

At the time I was teaching seminars for nurses through the Center for Health Awareness and had a traveling book-store that went with me. I sold the books I referred to in the seminar, or that I recommended. Why not sell Corkys, too? So, I ordered a box of twenty.

At the seminars I introduced Corky, told the story of how and why I got him, and offered them for sale. Over a period of several years, I probably sold at least 200 Corkys. Two hundred nurses took home anchors to a powerful weekend, and reminders that life can be fun and playful.

This was a potent demonstration for me of how some-thing that may seem like a negative can be a positive in the bigger picture. It was a sad thing to lose my original Corky, but that loss led to many happy moments for many people. I remember the joy on the faces of the two hundred nurses excited to have their own Corky. Corky has been an instru-ment to spread joy in the world.

I currently have a Corky in my bedroom where I see him every day. He has a bright red and blue outfit. His red nose has faded over the years, but he is smiling and sucking his thumb adorably. He still makes me smile whenever I look at him. And reminds me that there might be a silver lining in any bumps along my road.

Later
Building Blocks

I WAS TWENTY-FIVE YEARS old and naïve when I started my first post-graduate school job at Agnews State Hospital in San Jose, California. Ronald Reagan, the governor of California, had decided to close the state mental hospitals. My principal job as a psychiatric social worker was discharge planning for patients who were being released and had no home to return to. They weren't being released because they had been treated successfully and were well, but rather because the State decided to no longer care for them at the hospital.

My first assignment was on a locked ward of about 100 men who were all from the San Francisco area. I was frequently the only woman on the ward. I had a little office close to the nurses' station and I was often the only person on the ward not in uniform. The staff wore white; the patients wore khaki. The patients appreciated my business suits and dressy medium-heeled shoes, sometimes thanking me for dressing up for them. They said it made them feel like they still mattered. My door was always open and I was interested in any conversation that came my way.

The only time I remember being afraid was the first time Paulo tried to attack me when I entered the building. He thought I was his wife whom he hated. Fortunately, his

Huntington's chorea (inherited neurological disease) left him too uncoordinated to get to me. The other patients became very protective of me, and after that first incident, they would hold him back when I came in. Paulo couldn't navigate well enough to get to my office on his own.

Some of these men had been at Agnews for fifty years. Some had no family. Others had been disowned by family members. Clive had been hospitalized when he was nineteen following a football head injury. When I met him he was seventy, but he looked fifty, due to his protected life and lack of stress. Even though the ward was locked, Clive had full access to the grounds and often ran errands for staff between buildings. His sister, a prominent socialite in San Francisco, had told the world that her brother was dead. We had a letter on file from a past governor stating that Clive would never be able to leave the hospital. He was a gentle harmless man who spoke so little that I don't know if he wanted to leave or not. Like many of the patients, Clive didn't know life outside the hospital. While some were very comfortable there, they had nowhere to go, and didn't want to leave. They were being pushed out anyway. The State was opening Board and Care homes in the community to accommodate them, but the plans fell short of helping these men make the transition into a whole new way of living.

Another patient, Cecil, communicated very clearly that he didn't want to leave the cocoon that had protected him all these years. As part of the discharge planning, the patients had to have an income. For most of them, that meant applying for a State program called Aid to the Disabled.

I filled out the paperwork and they had to sign it. When Cecil refused to sign, the psychiatrist in charge of the ward put him in solitary confinement until he would sign it. It took about a week, but he eventually did. We placed him in a Board and Care home in San Francisco, and tragically, within a week he jumped off of a bridge and killed himself.

The world had changed since these men had lived in San Francisco fifty years ago. One of the psychiatric technicians and I took them in small groups on field trips to San Francisco to experience the new world they would be entering.

It was about an hour's drive from the hospital to The City. About ten minutes before arriving in San Francisco, the road curves around and the first view of the skyline is visible. Rounding that curve was the moment one of the men took off his hat and cried, moved by the sight of his old home. Others were anxious. We took them to lunch at a restaurant and LeRoy wet his pants while standing in a buffet line.

This was in the sixties, the days of the Flower Children in San Francisco. When we drove through Golden Gate Park, which was full of hippies, one of the men said "Those people seem crazier than we are," and he was right. We all had a good laugh over that.

Alan was a young patient who didn't clearly say he wanted to remain in the hospital, but his actions demonstrated it. His pattern was to go through the discharge planning, find a Board and Care home he felt comfortable with, and express excitement about leaving. Within a month of being out, he would set a fire, demonstrating that he was a danger to others and he would be back in Agnews. This happened several times before he told me he was scared out there and knew if he set a fire, he would get to come back where he felt safe.

Sidney had Cerebral Palsy. He was disfigured and had difficulty communicating. I learned to understand him, but it was a proficiency most people didn't take the time to develop. He was intelligent, and frustrated by his ineffective communication. He looked scary to strangers. Once, while he was in a park and had to go to the bathroom, someone saw him peeing in a bush and called the police. Fortunately, he was admitted to the State hospital instead of jail. He needed protection from others more than anyone needed protection from him.

Another patient, Jeremy, was a lawyer in his forties who believed aliens had implanted a device in his brain that gave him instructions he had to follow. Sometimes the voice told him to start fights with strangers. As we learned to know each other, he confided in me, with tears in his eyes, that he had to believe the alien story because the alternative was to admit that he was crazy.

Hans was a handsome, intelligent, German man who had been charged with killing his child. The court determined he wasn't of sound mind and needed to be hospitalized instead of standing trial. With great emotion he described to me what had happened. His young child had been in an accident, was dragged on the pavement, badly injured, and in great pain. He couldn't bear to witness his child in so much pain and did a mercy killing. He believed his actions had saved his child much needless suffering.

There were a number of patients admitted who'd flipped out on LSD at music festivals. Once they came down from the drug, they were pretty normal young men. By that time the long hair that had taken them years to grow had been forcibly cut off. This seemed to me more like punishment than treatment. Some of them were pretty angry, and I could understand why. My approach was to help them comprehend what society expected, and how they could alter their behavior in the future if they didn't want to be locked up again. This was a matter of learning who had authority and how they could protect themselves.

The line between sanity and insanity seemed fluid and capricious. Where anyone lands on that line depends on who gets to draw it. Dr. Yaminaka was the psychiatrist in charge of the ward during much of my Agnews stint. I often thought it would have been equally effective to give him the drugs instead of the patients. He was overweight, unhappy, and lacked empathy, patience, and understanding. He was obviously someone working in the wrong profession. I later learned that he committed suicide shortly after I left.

I had been obligated to work for the State for a year in exchange for a scholarship my second year of graduate school. I quit my job at Agnews State Hospital after fulfilling that one year commitment. I no longer wanted to watch the cruelty the patients were exposed to at the hands of the doctors and psychiatric technicians. The patients were being managed and controlled more than treated.

I took a six-week road trip across Canada with a friend and came back ready to find another job. My supervisor from Agnews called to invite me to return. I had been thinking about it a lot during my travels and was feeling like I had abandoned the patients. If they were being treated cruelly, they needed an advocate. I needed to make a decision about working there, not based on what was comfortable for me, but on where I could be of the most benefit. I went back and worked there two more years, listening to patients and advocating for their human rights and dignity.

CHAPTER THIRTEEN
MARRIAGE

In the Mennonite community I was raised in, if a woman wasn't at least engaged by age twenty-one, she was on her way to being an old maid, and that was a fate worse than death. I worried about that in my youth, but as I started experiencing adventures out in the real world, and my values and beliefs evolved, I decided I wanted to get married when I was thirty. I wanted time to have a career and explore the world before I committed to a lifetime of togetherness.

When I was twenty-nine, I met Bob through the Sierra Club. He had been on a Sierra Club trip over Memorial Day in which four people died in an avalanche. I'd been dating one of the men who died in the accident. The Sierra Club organized a memorial service for the four who died. Bob and I met at a meeting of the group of Sierra Clubbers planning that memorial service.

For me, the death of my friend demonstrated the fragility of life, and the importance of seizing the moment. I was attracted to Bob right away, and took the initiative to ask him out for coffee. I later found out he wouldn't have approached me because he wanted to respect the loss I'd just experienced. He didn't know that I'd only had a few dates with the man who was killed and although this was a traumatic loss, it wasn't as distressing as it would have been if we'd been long-term partners.

Bob and I were initially drawn to each other by our mutual interest in nature, the mountains, and in building a house in the mountains. We were both excited to meet someone with whom we could follow that dream. We purchased mountain property before officially becoming engaged. Our mountain property was part of Las Cumbres Conservation Corporation in the Santa Cruz Mountains of California. Our property had a view of Monterey Bay which was twenty miles away, with a sunset view 365 days a year. It was beautiful and wild.

One hundred twenty families had purchased 1200 acres and created a planned development in which each house was built on less than 1 acre, with over 1,000 acres of wild land with trails for exploring. We built our own roads, had our own water company, our own volunteer fire department, and regular community meetings. Being part of such a community was another dream come true.

We spent many weekends clearing our property. The person who had owned it before us had landed in the hospital after starting to clear the land, burning brush that was full of poison oak. His lungs were filled with poison oak smoke and he was very sick. We learned from him, and were very careful in our clearing process. We rented a wood chipper instead of burning anything.

Somewhere during this process, we got married. In retrospect, I can recognize that we had a "hippie" wedding. We got married outside on the lawn of the house a group of us were renting on a one-quarter acre property with a creek running through it. This was a beautiful outdoor setting. My friend Joan made my wedding dress that was white dotted Swiss fabric with purple trim. Bob wore purple velvet pants and a blousy white silk shirt. We both had long hair and I exerted great effort to straighten mine.

Fifty close friends and family attended the ceremony. My parents were both there even though they had been divorced for several years. My father walked me down the driveway from our house to the wedding site while a classical guitarist played part of the Joaquin Rodrigo concerto. My Grandfather offered a prayer. My friend Gail sang "The First Time Ever I Saw Your Face" (made popular by Roberta Flack). An ex-boyfriend, who was an Episcopalian minister, performed the ceremony. One of my prior roommates and his boyfriend catered the affair. It was an extraordinary day, full of love and connection.

Bob was an electrical engineer, an inventor, and the most self-confident person I'd ever met. He was good at solving problems, fixing things, and believed he could build a house from reading books about the process. Even though he had no experience, neither one of us ever doubted that he could do it.

We designed our house together, but in order to get a construction loan, we needed a licensed contractor. Lending institutions didn't have the confidence in Bob that I did. We paid a contractor $500 to sign his name to our documents and he visited the construction site to be sure we knew what we were doing. The twentieth lending institution I approached finally gave us our construction loan.

We borrowed a 19-foot mobile home from some friends, moved it onto the property, and lived in it while we started construction. Bob, who is six feet, two inches tall, couldn't stand up straight in the mobile home, but he spent so little time in there, it didn't matter.

Bob quit his engineering job to work full time on building the house. I worked as a psychiatric social worker for Santa Clara County Mental Health Department half time, and did what I could to help build the house with him. I took woodshop classes at the local high school and learned how to use tools and build furniture. I learned how to hang, tape, and texture dry wall. I learned how to wire electrical fixtures. I learned how to lay tile and built a tiled bathtub and shower. I learned how to do leaded glass and made a hanging Tiffany lamp for our dining room. I made all the drapes for our house on my mother's old treadle sewing machine. This was a busy, creative, happy time.

While we were building the house, I had a recurring dream that there was a problem with the foundation. This was a disturbing dream, but I couldn't figure out what it meant. It wasn't until we had mostly finished the house and birthed our child in the house that I realized the foundation that had a problem was the relationship between Bob and me. The glue that held us together was the goal and activity of finding our land and creating our community and our home. Once the bulk of that task was done and we examined our relationship for the passion we each desired for a happy life, we couldn't find it. We did find a therapist and my hope was that we could repair our foundation, but Bob found passion elsewhere. That's the subject of another chapter.

CHAPTER FOURTEEN
HOME BIRTH

BOB AND I HAD BEEN married about three years. After weathering the stress of building a house together, even though it wasn't finished, we had created enough of a nest that we were eager to start a family.

On the nurture versus nature question, we wanted to make sure the nature part was covered in our planning. Not knowing when a soul enters the new body, we chose to conceive our child at Tassajara Hot Springs, a Zen monastery with a summer guest season that was an annual vacation spot for us. Any soul hanging around there would be wise, loving, and patient.

On a hot afternoon in July of 1975, in our little Tassajara rustic wood cabin, I could feel that life had begun inside my body. If the soul entered the body at conception, in nine months we would be living with a wise old Buddhist soul. But what if the soul joined the body at birth? We couldn't take the chance of having that happen in a hospital where the energy is frantic and there could be desperate fearful souls hanging around. Could we have a home birth?

The house we had built was on a beautiful mountain ridge with a view of Monterey Bay that was twenty miles away. We were surrounded by nature and wild life. I could be face-to-face with a deer through the kitchen window.

Sitting on our deck I could feel the wind from a vulture soaring by. With no traffic noise, no airplanes, and no neighbors within earshot, the quiet was palpable. We were sure only a loving soul would enter that peaceful world.

But would it be safe? I was thirty-four years old and our mountain home was a forty-five-minute drive from the nearest hospital. What if something went wrong? Could I risk my life and the life of my child because of what many people would call a foolish idea? Bob was all for a home birth, but this felt like it had to be my decision. I needed to be comfortable with it.

I found a doctor who attended home births, but he wouldn't take me on unless I severed my association with my regular OB/GYN doctor. There was something about the home birth doctor that felt creepy, and I loved my doctor, even though he was adamant that a home birth was dangerous for me. Then I met Judy, a lay midwife. As I spent several hours talking to her about the pros and cons, I could feel my body relax into trusting her. My intuition told me I could safely have a home birth if Judy were present.

On April 7th, while shopping for groceries, I started having contractions in the produce section of the grocery store. I called Bob and headed home. We called Judy, my friend Georgia, and Bob's sister Carolyn, who had agreed to be there. Everyone showed up. Judy brought two women she was training to be midwives, and the big event began.

It was a stormy night with hard rain and fierce winds, but my focus was on what was happening in my body. I had prepared for this moment for nine months. I had learned how to breathe with the contractions, how to relax, but I didn't expect the level of pain I experienced. I was in it for the end result. Did I really have to go through this process? I kept thinking about the millions of women who had done this before me, and I gathered strength from them. There was no way out but through this portal.

After about ten hours of labor, Judy said it seemed like I was stuck and she didn't feel comfortable continuing to wait. She wanted us to go to the hospital. Everyone started packing up what we needed and getting ready to go. I was suddenly left in the "birth" room alone. I started imagining walking down the stairs to the car so we could leave, and I didn't think I could make it. The urge to push became the most compelling feeling I had ever encountered. I started making guttural sounds that I hadn't heard come out of my mouth before. Judy heard me from the other room and rushed in. She loudly announced that the baby was coming, and started bossing everyone around. Within the hour, I was looking into the beautiful eyes of our son, Brian.

Carolyn had been given the task of documenting the event with her camera. She took lots of pictures of me in distress during those ten hours of labor, but during the last hour she was so captivated with watching the miracle of a new human being enter the world that she forgot her job. Even without any visual documentation, the memory of my experience is vivid enough to firmly position it as the most profound of my life.

Years later, when Brian was in his late twenties, he announced he was going to Tassajara Hot Springs for a six-week student work-study experience. He had been to

Tassajara for short visits as a child, but hadn't visited it for many years. We hadn't told him about our planning his conception and wondering when the soul enters the body. When he returned from that six-week stretch, he came back a serious meditator, and settled the question. He's definitely a wise old Buddhist soul.

CHAPTER FIFTEEN

LOSS

BRIAN IS ALMOST TWO. BOB and I have realized our dreams of building our mountain house, and starting our family. We are struggling in our relationship, wondering what's next. Bob has gone back to full-time employment as an electrical engineer and works on completing the house evenings and weekends. I'm employed ten hours a week at the County Mental Health Center, and spend most of my time mothering Brian and working on house-finishing projects.

Bob is an engineer and good at fixing and building things. I am a psychiatric social worker who loves talking about and processing feelings. Once our projects are completed, it seems we don't have much in common.

One evening, after a session with our therapist, Bob and I had what I thought was the most meaningful conversation we had had—maybe ever. We talked about how we felt about the therapy session, each other, and our future. We shared deep feelings. At the end of the conversation, Bob asked me if this is what I had been wanting. I excitedly said "yes," to which he responded, "This is the most boring conversation I have ever had and I hope we never have to do it again." I was stunned. How could anyone not enjoy sharing feelings with someone they loved? Now I was seriously pessimistic about our future together.

When Bob came home from work one day and told me he had agreed to go to a Scientology workshop with his friend, I cried. I had a sinking feeling that this would lead to no good. Bruce had been trying to talk both of us into exploring Scientology for several months, and I was distraught that Bob was going for it. Even though I wasn't optimistic about "us," I was still hopeful. It felt like Scientology would be the last straw in pulling us in different directions.

Within a few months, Bob declared that Scientology had changed his world view so much that he couldn't be in relationship with someone who wasn't a Scientologist. If I wanted our marriage to survive, I had to be open to the possibility of becoming a Scientologist. I signed up for the Communications course.

The theory undergirding Scientology was compelling. We are thetans (souls) who may have lived before. All of our life experiences have created grooves in our psyches that influence who we are today. Current situations in our lives may elicit a reaction that is overblown because we are reacting to other grooves that already exist from previous events. These previous grooves may be so powerful that they prevent us from responding to something wholly in the present. There was nothing in these concepts that I disagreed with, yet I didn't feel at ease in the Scientology world. Everything felt too black and white, not leaving the option of being human.

The Communications course had some exciting moments. When I was looking deeply into the eyes of another student, I felt a connection at a soul/energy level that I hadn't experienced before; I thought there may be something to this. So, I signed up for auditing, a process used to eliminate the grooves from past experiences by reliving them until the "charge" is gone. Auditors measured "charge" with an e-meter (measured electro dermal activity) that was hooked up to the tin cans I held in my hands. We would start by talking about a current situation and then review and relive earlier similar situations until the "charge" no longer registered. The goal was to become "Clear," thus able to respond to any current situation without reacting to past traumatic events.

During the time I was doing this auditing process, I had a cold. As long as I had the cold, the cold was all I was allowed to work on in the auditing sessions. These sessions weren't cheap. After spending hundreds of dollars dealing with the cold, I was motivated to get rid of it. Based on my past experiences with imagery, I imagined an army of little men with mini-vacuum cleaners cleaning out my sinuses. A few days of this practice and my cold was gone.

In my next auditing session, the auditor was ready to work on the cold again. I told him the cold was gone and I was ready to progress forward with my auditing. He asked how I had gotten rid of the cold. When I told him what I had done, he said I wasn't advanced enough to do that. Based on his belief, he was willing to work only on my cold in the auditing session.

By that time, I had had a few other experiences that made me question moving forward with Scientology. It was a perfect fit for Bob who was an engineer not comfortable with emotions. But I was a psychiatric social worker who savored the messiness of emotions. I resisted any attempt to mold me into what I perceived as robot-like.

This auditing fiasco was the last straw for me. We had paid a lot of money to Scientology in advance for my services, and I had used only a small portion of it. I wanted my money back. I quickly learned that money goes only one way in Scientology exchanges. They brought out the big guns and sent me to the ethics officer to convince me to stay. His hard sell made me even more anxious to put Scientology behind me. When they couldn't convince me to stay, they persuaded Bob to pay me cash for my unused services, and he used the credit for his own auditing.

In the same time period, Barbie, a staff member from the Scientology headquarters in Florida, was tasked with evaluating the effectiveness of the San Jose Scientology organization. In order to do that, she met with each of the students receiving their services. When I had my fifteen-minute appointment with her, I had the same feeling I did when Bob said he was taking a Scientology course. A sinking feeling that this would lead to no good. Bob also had a fifteen-minute meeting with Barbie that day. He came home that night and said he wanted a divorce. His main criteria for a partner was that she share his passion for Scientology. He had met that person in Barbie. That was July 31st.

My plate was already full of emotions because my mother was in the process of dying. She had fallen and broken her hip. She had surgery, but her heart was not strong enough for her to recover. She was in a care facility in Reedley, the same little town where I was born. I had visited her in July, but once our divorce was on the table, even though I received phone calls telling me she was dying, I chose not to visit her again. She loved Bob, and I knew I couldn't visit her without telling her about our divorce. I was concerned that her worry about my future might make it more difficult for her to let go. I wanted her to be able to die believing that I was happily married and being cared for by Bob. One of the biggest regrets in my life is not being with my mother when she died.

She died on August 23rd. By that time Bob was traveling to spend weekends with Barbie and had essentially left our marriage. He didn't go with me to my mother's funeral, leaving me with the task of explaining his absence to my Mennonite relatives.

On the night I returned home from my mother's funeral, Bob knocked on my bedroom door. We were sleeping in separate bedrooms by that time. He asked if we could talk. I said yes, thinking he might want to know about the funeral, how I was feeling, or offer his sympathy. I was sad and vulnerable, needing some support. My need overrode my clear thinking of what Bob was capable of. He didn't ask any questions about how the funeral was or how I was. He wanted to talk about Brian. He chose that moment to tell me that he was going to do everything in his power to get custody of Brian. I couldn't believe he was telling me this, especially at this particular time. I told myself that I should remember this moment; I would be a fool to ever again expect any emotional support from Bob.

On September 1st, Brian and I and our cat, Clyde,

moved out of our mountain home into a condominium in what we called the "flatlands." As a single mother, I didn't want to stay in the mountains, forty-five minutes from civilization. Besides, the house felt more like Bob's than mine since he had quit his job and spent almost a year actually building it.

Bob went to visit Barbie the weekend I moved, but let me use his truck to move. Friends (all women) helped me. On the last trip down the hill that night, Brian was in the passenger seat with his favorite blanket that was his constant source of comfort. Clyde the cat was on the floor at Brian's feet. Driving down the curvy mountainous road, Clyde vomited all over Brian's blanket. Clyde was expressing what I felt. This was a nauseating situation.

It was late. We were stressed and exhausted, but Brian couldn't go to sleep without his blanket. There was a laundry room in the building. I had to find quarters and wash and dry the blanket before we could go to bed. What a way to start on our new adventure; it could only get easier from here.

Shortly after I moved out, Bob asked me to have lunch with him near the office where I worked. He had something he wanted to talk to me about. Even though I had learned not to expect any emotional support from him, I was still surprised by the subject of that lunch conversation. He invited me to his wedding. He said I was important to him and he wanted me to be there. He had gotten a Mexican divorce and was marrying Barbie six weeks after I moved out, in the house he and I had built. I cried and let him know that would be much too painful for me.

They lived in our mountain house for twenty years before Bob divorced her. Losing the marriage and our mountain home was a dark night for me, leading to a transformation and a new career.

CHAPTER SIXTEEN

CENTER FOR HEALTH AWARENESS

THE INCOME FROM WORKING TEN hours a week for the Santa Clara County Mental Health Department as a psychiatric social worker was enough when we were married and had another income in the household. But now, life had changed and I needed to increase my income. I had some alimony for a few months, but needed to figure out a different strategy soon.

I was feeling burned-out in the social work world and hoped applying my skills to the business world would create new challenges and interest. I applied for many jobs. While I was being told I was either over or under qualified for all of them, I took a personal growth program called *Adventures in Attitudes* that opened up a whole new world for me.

Adventures in Attitudes (AIA) was a thirty-hour personal growth program created by Personal Dynamics, a company in Minneapolis, and done through network marketing. Cathy (a nurse I worked with at the County Mental Health Department) had taken the training and I'd overheard her talking about it in the next cubicle at work. This program sounded like just what I needed to add some excitement and direction to my new life.

I took the weekend training which included certifying

me to become a facilitator of the course. Not only did this course create a new career for me, it also introduced me to a whole new way of experiencing the world. It introduced me to the power of my subconscious mind. I started reading books on the subject and attended a New Thought church. I felt like I had a new strategy for having some control over my destiny.

I immersed myself in learning about Prosperity Consciousness. Besides reading books, I listened to tapes anytime I was in my car (in the late seventies, before CDs existed), I did the exercises, and I sent ten percent of my income to the author of the tapes. This was to demonstrate that I truly believed I had enough and my supply was unlimited. I started carrying a $100 bill in my purse so I would never be broke. In four months, I quadrupled my income by using the principles I'd learned in AIA and in the Prosperity Consciousness training. It worked.

Cathy and I were teaching AIA for Continuing Education for nurses. This was at a time when nurses were first required to have thirty hours of CEs every two years. They could meet that requirement in a weekend by taking our course. We purchased mailing lists, sent out brochures, and filled up our classes. Our success with AIA not only created an income for us, it also led to free trips to Hawaii and the Bahamas. We were often the top salespeople in the Personal Dynamics organization and were awarded free trips to the annual conferences.

We formed a non-profit organization, The Center for Health Awareness, a holistic health center as well as a vehicle to support our educational endeavors. We purchased a building to accommodate our needs, and also rented out office space to practitioners, including a holistic MD who was there one day a week, several massage therapists, a Rolfer, a Chinese Herbologist, and several therapists. Our hope was that they'd work together, treating patients holistically. The reality was that they each believed what they offered was what a patient most needed, and they didn't collaborate with each other. Our dream of the holistic health center didn't materialize as we imagined, but we had much success with our educational programs.

In teaching AIA, we had to purchase materials from the Personal Dynamics organization. This was a big chunk of our costs. After several years and increasing success, we designed our own thirty-hour program, *The Turning Point*. More income for us. At the height of our success, we had eleven trainers teaching our program around the country; we owned the building that housed The Center for Health Awareness; and we owned the printing press that printed our materials. Life was good.

Then the Continuing Education market changed. Hospitals started providing it for their nurses, and our seminars no longer filled up. We needed to shift our business model, but we couldn't agree on how to do that. As our finances dwindled, I lowered my salary and pleaded with Cathy to lower hers, but she refused. I felt like I couldn't work with her anymore. I wanted Cathy to quit and let me run the business because I was convinced I could turn it around, but she refused.

I developed pneumonia and as part of my healing process, I went to Santa Fe, New Mexico, to work with a healer who also introduced me to a Guatemalan shaman. In a sunrise session in the shaman's tent on a mountain top, with rattles and feathers and dancing, the shaman told me that my job was killing me and if I wanted to heal, I had to quit doing what I was doing. He also said the people I was working with were sapping my energy. My intuition agreed with this, and it was a relief to have an outside source tell me it was time to move on.

I left the Center for Health Awareness, and six months later Cathy bankrupted it. This created a crisis in belief for me. We had been teaching that we created our own reality, yet Cathy and I were not able to demonstrate what we were teaching. We wanted our business to succeed, but we weren't able to make it happen. I felt disillusioned and discouraged.

My decision to leave The Center also left me with no meaningful work, no income, and a huge blank slate upon which I would write the next chapter of my life.

CHAPTER SEVENTEEN

ABORTION OR MISCARRIAGE

BEFORE LEAVING THE CENTER FOR Health Awareness, I met Michael. A friend attended a weekend workshop called Integrity Training. She stayed at my house for the weekend and came home from the workshop saying there was a man she thought I should meet. I went to her graduation on Sunday night and met Michael, a handsome, smooth, charming man, eleven years younger than me.

Our first connection was around the Japanese Martial art called Aikido, which Michael was studying. Cathy and I were using Aikido in our workshop as a metaphor for dealing with potentially harmful energy by diverting it back to the person sending it. Although I'd read about Aikido and seen movies about it, I hadn't actually experienced it. Michael invited me to visit one of his Aikido classes.

We made a plan for me to visit the class the following week. The day before the planned visit, Michael showed up at my office to tell me he had to take an unexpected trip and needed to cancel. I invited him in for a cup of tea. I didn't know at the time he was nervous about the trip he was taking the following day. He told me later that the cup of tea and my calming presence had made a big difference for him, and impressed him.

While he was gone, I had bladder surgery to repair the

leakage I'd experienced after childbirth. Our first "date," after his trip and my surgery, was going to church together on Christmas Eve. He accompanied me to the New Thought church I was attending for a candlelight service. I was still catheterized on that date with a bag hidden in my pants leg.

Because of my surgery, I was prohibited from any sexual activity for six weeks. The timing of that surgery coinciding with meeting Michael was profound in starting our relationship. Michael was used to acting much faster than that. He had had many short-term relationships and was pictured and advertised in a local singles paper as a desirable and confirmed bachelor. Because of the timing of my surgery, he was forced to slow down with me. By the time we could be sexual, we had spent a lot of time together, connecting and bonding emotionally. We were falling in love.

We had been dating only a couple of months when I got pregnant. I was forty-five years old and thought I was past my child-bearing years so I was not as careful as I could have been. We agreed that the relationship was too new for us to solidify it with a child. I saw my gynecologist and made an appointment to have an abortion.

The night before the scheduled abortion, I thought about the being growing inside of me, and what my values were. The Mennonites who raised me were pacifists. The men in our family were conscientious objectors. In my heart I was a pacifist and couldn't go through with what felt like killing another being.

In my imagination, I had a conversation with the being. I told him/her that this wasn't a good time in my life to have a child. I said the relationship with Michael was new and I didn't know how long it would last. Even if it lasted a long time, Michael and I needed more time to develop our relationship before we could focus our energy on raising a child. I said I couldn't make the decision to terminate the pregnancy, but I trusted the being to decide if it would come into this situation that wasn't ideal. I made it clear that my preference was for the pregnancy not to continue.

I went to sleep and was awakened by cramping a few hours later. I went to the bathroom and expelled a bloody mass into the toilet. Could this be the fetus? Could my conversation have caused it to abort naturally? I was in awe that this miracle could have actually happened. I wanted to be sure, so I managed to carefully save what I could in a clean glass jar and took it the next day to my appointment with the gynecologist. She confirmed that it was the fetus that had aborted itself. I learned this spontaneous abortion was called a miscarriage.

Losing this child didn't feel like a loss to me and I had no sadness about it. Besides being a huge relief, this was also a strong lesson for me about trusting both my body and the unseen world. This felt like a miracle, yet also felt natural. This is how life should work.*

---

* I have since learned of the work of Gladys Taylor McGarey, MD, who has been described as the mother of holistic medicine. She believed "that the soul coming in is a conscious human being, and as such, has choices and these choices are real even before the conscious mind knows that it is making choices. These are choices made at a soul level." In her approach to pregnant women who were considering abortion, she suggested they talk to the baby. She said more than half the time the pregnancy aborted spontaneously. (The Choice for Pregnancy, by Gladys McGarey, published in Women's Wellness, July/August 2006).

CHAPTER EIGHTEEN
A MOTHER'S DILEMMA

As an only child, I felt cheated. I cut kids' pictures out of magazines and pretended they were my brothers or sisters. I swore I would never have an only child. I wanted to give my child the brother or sister I had always craved. When my first husband and I separated, Brian was two. I wasn't willing to have another child as a single parent. Not only was Brian deprived of a brother or sister, he was living with only one parent.

At the time of our separation, Brian's father said he was going to do everything he could to get custody of Brian. Fortunately, he wasn't proactive enough to actually do anything about that, but his threat worried me. Mothering Brian was the best thing that had ever happened to me. He was an incredibly sweet and intelligent child, and filled my life with abundant joy. Even though single parenting wasn't easy, I couldn't imagine life without Brian. We had years of laughter and connection that fed my soul.

The happiest time of my life was the first years of mothering Brian. Of course, the birth itself was a miracle. An actual person came out of my body. His body was so perfectly formed, and his eyes "pierced my soul" from the first minute he came out. And then there were the moments of breast feeding with those eyes gazing into mine. I had never experienced such a bond with another being. I have also never experienced the depth of despair and anger that he brought out in me. I understood child abuse in a way I never could have without being a parent. Kahlil Gibran was right when he said the depth of your negative feelings will equal the height of your joy. Both extremes were there with parenthood. When he cried and couldn't be comforted by any of the strategies that had worked in the past, I wanted to throw him out the window so I wouldn't have to hear his pain. I've never felt so helpless, or so angry.

Watching him learn to navigate the world—to talk, to walk, and to laugh—was bliss. His delight was contagious. Watching him gleefully follow Clyde, the cat, around the house in his walker was pure joy.

When he was just learning to talk, his godfather came over for dinner and was so impressed with Brian's vocabulary that he was picking up things on the table and saying, "What's this, Brian?" Brian named the salt, a spoon, a glass, and finally Brian picked up the ketchup and said, "What's this, John?" He could play that game, too.

As Brian got older, parenting became more challenging. By the time he was ten, I was feeling less and less competent as a parent. Even though a boy his age lived right next door, Brian refused to play with him. He was isolating in our house and I couldn't get him out. We had fights that ended with him going into his room, slamming the door, and not coming out for hours. Our communication channels were crumbling. I wondered if having daily access to his father as a role model would help.

His father and his current wife had wanted Brian to

come live with them since they'd married seven years before, but I felt Brian needed the nurturing he was getting from me. I also hadn't wanted to send Brian to live in a Scientology household. Both his father and his wife were heavily into Scientology. Now that Brian was ten, and I was feeling desperate and inadequate as a parent, I hoped he had developed his personality and his values enough that he wouldn't be swallowed up into Scientology.

They had two other children so Brian would get to be part of an intact family. They were living in the house where Brian was born and they had plenty of room for him. I thought there was also plenty of love in that household and Brian would thrive.

I had also just lost the Center for Health Awareness, the business that had supported us for the past seven years, so I was without an income and unable to pay the mortgage on the house I had purchased for us five years before. I rented it out and moved into an apartment with the man who later became my second husband. I was feeling depleted, discouraged, and lost. At least Brian would have a stable home and family.

Letting Brian go live with his dad may be the hardest thing I've ever done. I believed it would give Brian the best life and I was doing it for his benefit, but there was a part of me that labeled myself a bad mother. Brian didn't want to live there and I felt like I was abandoning him. We also had to give away his dog since his dad wanted to protect the deer around their mountain home. The day Chewy was picked up by the new owners was the last time I saw Brian cry.

Brian lived with his father and his family, sharing a room with his half-brother, for the next seven years, until he went to college. We spent many weekends, vacations, and holidays together and still had some good times, but our relationship felt strained. I felt like he was holding a grudge, still mad at me for abandoning him. My attempts to talk about this with him were futile until recently.

A few months ago, I asked him some direct questions and listened to his answers without defending myself. He told me how awful his life was living at his dad's house. He said his stepmother was angry all the time; she treated him differently than her two kids. Her two kids had a close relationship with each other and he felt left out and very much alone. They lived far from any neighbors so he had no one else to play with or talk to. He said he tried to tell me how bad it was while it was happening, but I couldn't hear him. He said this experience has formed who he is today – a loner who doesn't want to get married or have kids.

When I asked directly if he was still mad at me for sending him to live with his dad, he said, "I wish it had never happened." I told him through my tears that I was very sorry and I also wish it had never happened. I made several decisions during that time period that I regret today.

As I write this, Brian is forty-five years old and has recently moved to Portland, the same town where his half-brother lives. They have a warm relationship which I don't think would have happened if they hadn't shared a bedroom for seven years. And I've recently gotten to observe the close relationship he has with his father.

His father had emergency major heart surgery last

year while he was visiting and working in California. He couldn't return to his home in Hawaii because he couldn't fly post-surgery, so he needed somewhere to stay and be cared for after ten days in the hospital. He and his third wife were in the process of divorce, so he was alone.

His sister and I went to visit him in the hospital, and it was her idea that he come stay with me as he recovered. We had become better friends during the twenty years he had been with wife number three. I lived alone in a three-bedroom house, so there was a bedroom and bathroom for him. I felt comfortable with the plan.

I picked Brian up at the Sacramento airport the evening of October 15th. The next day his dad was being released from the hospital in San Jose, two hours away. I had an important doctor's appointment and couldn't go pick him up. A friend took me to my appointment while Brian drove my car to San Jose and picked up his dad. They got to my house around six p.m. and I had dinner ready. As the three of us sat at the dinner table together, we marveled that this was the first time in 42 years that we had been together as a family of three.

I was incredibly grateful that Brian came from Portland and took care of his dad for the first week he was with me. In the beginning, Bob couldn't do much for himself. Brian helped him shower and dress, and took him out for walks every morning. He was weak from the surgery. If I had been the helper walking with him, and he fell, I wouldn't have been able to do much with his six foot, two-inch tall body. Brian is equally tall, and strong. The first day their walk was to the driveway and back.

Each day they went a little further. By the time Brian had to leave, the fear of falling was no longer an issue. After ten weeks, he was pretty much back to normal and was able to fly home to Hawaii.

It warmed my heart to see the tenderness, humor, and compassion that Brian demonstrated toward his father. It was a week of healing to have the three of us living together for the first time since we'd separated when Brian was two.

I've heard the theory that breast cancer in the left breast has to do with a mother/child relationship. My breast cancer diagnosis in my left breast was three years after I let Brian go live with his dad. Even though Brian and I have both said we wished it hadn't happened, we accept that it did. The events of the past have helped form who he is today, and we both like the person he's become.

My challenge now is to forgive myself and let go of the belief that my decision made me a bad mother. I've worked on this in workshops and in therapy, but it's not done. I have an intellectual acceptance and understanding that I was doing the best with what I knew and who I was at the time. But the emotional angst and regret are still just below the surface.

CHAPTER NINETEEN

POLYAMORY

I HAD NEVER HEARD OF Polyamory before Michael imposed it on our marriage. Theoretically, it sounded like a good idea. Who doesn't want more love in the world? I believe we are all connected and Oneness is the ideal. I wondered if polyamory could be a vehicle to get there.

Polyamory is defined as "the practice of engaging in multiple romantic (and typically sexual) relationships, with the consent of all the people involved." It's different than an open marriage where each person can have other relationships outside of the marriage. It's different from Swinging because it involves love, connection, and long-term relationships. Polyamory, as Michael wanted to practice it, involved us having connections with other couples together.

In an effort to save our marriage, I agreed to try it. It reminded me of trying to be a Scientologist to save my first marriage. I again was trying to mold myself to fit the needs of my husband. I learned again that doesn't work. But I went through several traumatic years before I acknowledged that it didn't work for me. I needed to leave a very stressful situation to save my life. Saving my life became more important than saving the marriage.

We met a couple, Mauricio and Olivia, at a Tantra workshop. They were intelligent, good-looking, successful, and attracted to us. We spent several weekends together, one at their home in San Diego, and one at our home in Santa Cruz. Michael was in ecstasy. I was in hell.

We learned they were part of a triad with another woman. At first Olivia had been resistant to the idea, but she had warmed up to it and now she and Mauricio and Pat were a threesome who all loved each other. They seemed very comfortable doing things as any combination of two-somes or a threesome. They assured me that I would get over my resistance just like Olivia had, and the five of us would be happy together.

Pat came to spend a few days with Michael and me at our home in Santa Cruz. She felt like her "family" was being threatened and she wanted to get to know Michael and me to discern if we were a good fit to be included in their group. I liked Pat. In any other circumstance, we might have been able to be friends. While Pat was ready to include us, I was resistant to joining this unconventional "family."

As part of the process of recruiting me, the five of us had dinner together in San Francisco. To me, it felt like four against one. I didn't feel like anyone was on my side. They were all feeling the glow of the honeymoon phase of this new relationship and were telling me how wonderful it was. I felt like I had accidentally landed on another planet where nobody spoke my language. But I was still trying to be open to new possibilities.

Another part of their plan that night was for Olivia, Michael, and me to spend the night together in a hotel to assist me in overcoming any jealousy, and learning to know Olivia better. This may have been the worst night of my life. Michael slept between us in a king size bed. When I awoke during the night and his back was to me as he was snuggling with her, I felt like someone was tearing my heart out and shredding it. I wanted to scream, cry, and get out of the situation. I was trapped. I didn't have a car in San Francisco and didn't feel like I could leave. The only thing I could do was cry and comfort myself like I did when I was locked in the closet at age three. This night didn't help me overcome my jealousy. Instead, it triggered me to fully feel the betrayal and the jealousy that came with it. This was not what I signed up for when I married Michael.

After that night, I made a decision not to participate in this polyamorous world, but Michael was hooked. He and Olivia had bonded and wanted to continue their relationship. The five of us had planned a two-week trip to Mexico, including one week at a Tantra workshop in Tulum. I decided not to go. They all wanted me to join them, but I had no interest in even one more night of what I had experienced in the San Francisco hotel room. Two weeks sounded like torture. The four of them went and said they had a wonderful time, while I sat with the question of what I could do to minimize the pain of Michael's lifestyle choice.

In the beginning of this exploration into Polyamory, we attended a "Loving More" conference at Harbin Hot Springs. There were several hundred people there embracing the Polyamory lifestyle. I got several surprises, in addition to an introduction to the polyamorous community. I was surprised to see a friend from my home town that I wouldn't have guessed was involved in this community. I think she was equally surprised to see me. I learned that people who are in this community know it is out of the norm and they don't talk about it outside of the community.

Another surprise happened when I was in the dining hall that weekend, in line to get my food. I noticed two women sitting at a table who seemed to be staring at me. One of them had the tell-tale turban on her head and looked like a cancer patient. The other younger one approached me. After verifying that I was Jan Adrian, she asked if I would come talk to her mother. Her mother was a cancer patient and had recently attended one of my *Cancer as a Turning Point*™ conferences.

She seemed relieved to have my ear all to herself (her daughter went somewhere else to give us privacy). She told me she was there that weekend with her boyfriend who was trying to engage her in the world of polyamory. She didn't want to share her boyfriend with other women, and had no interest in polyamory. She said she had advanced cancer and had lost her motivation to fight it. She said, "If I get better from cancer, I will still have to deal with my boyfriend's interest in polyamory and that feels more stressful than dying from cancer."

She died about two weeks later.

That meeting left me with the question for myself—would I rather die than deal with the stress of polyamory? I was dealing with cancer too, and I know stress feeds cancer. There was another option for me. I could leave the marriage. Would I rather die than live without Michael?

That dichotomy wasn't clear to me at the time. I was very much in love with Michael and I clung to the hope that I could make it work somehow.

It took a final-straw incident for me to acknowledge the dichotomy and make the painstaking decision to leave the marriage. I had told Michael I didn't want to participate in his polyamory world, but I was willing to accompany him to workshops as long as our sexual activity was limited to the two of us. At one of these events, we met Clarice. I watched them dancing together and noticed that there seemed to be an attraction between them.

After this weekend event, Michael was leaving directly for Southern California for a week of helicopter training. I took him to the airport on my way home. We talked about his attraction to Clarice and we agreed that we would discuss it more fully when he returned from the week in Southern California.

We talked on the phone every night during that training and it wasn't until he got home that he told me Clarice was there with him. They stayed in a hotel together and had unprotected sex, something he had promised me he wouldn't do with anyone. That was the final straw. When he told me that, I said I couldn't do this anymore. I couldn't embrace his lifestyle; I couldn't trust him. I wanted a divorce.

Shortly after that I had a recurrence of my breast cancer on the left side and simultaneously had a new cancer in the right breast. I had read the theory that cancer in the right breast had to do with a partner relationship. Bingo again. This was in 2002. The message was loud and clear.

Staying in this marriage felt like the same as choosing death. I chose life and had a husbandectomy.

Turning
Points

CHAPTER TWENTY

LEARNING TO DANCE

WHEN DANCING WAS THE SPORT being taught in junior high school gym class, I had a note from my minister excusing me from class. Dancing wasn't allowed in the Mennonite Brethren church, another form of expression that most of the world had access to, but was forbidden in my world. I didn't question it at the time. If I had questioned it, I probably would have been told that dancing could lead to sex, and of course sex was not allowed outside of marriage.

Most of my friends and all my family were entrenched in the evangelical Christian world where dancing was a sin, so I didn't know anyone who danced. There were two other girls in my gym class with notes from their ministers, one from a Baptist church and one from the Church of Christ. The three of us played ping-pong during gym class and became good friends.

As I grew into adulthood and eventually left the Mennonite world behind, I felt like everyone else knew something I didn't know. I felt left out and different. I wanted to fit in. I wanted to learn how to dance.

When I was thirty-nine, I took myself to an Arthur Murray Dance studio for dancing lessons, with the goal of coming out as a dancer on my 40th birthday. I took individual lessons, and went to weekly group lessons where I got to dance with other students. I also dated one of the instructors and got some good practice out in the world. I learned the difference between a Waltz, a Foxtrot, East Coast Swing, West Coast Swing, Rhumba, and Cha-Cha.

I prepared for months for my 40th birthday, and it was a joyous occasion. About thirty of my friends were seated at tables in a U-shape in the hall I rented. In the middle of the U was a dance floor. I'd hired a Middle Eastern caterer who served delicious food. And then the fun began.

I had asked each person invited to offer some kind of entertainment that evening. Greg played his guitar and sang a ballad. Arlene read a poem she had written. The grand finale was me dancing the Rhumba with my dancing instructor from Arthur Murray. He had choreographed a Rhumba to *Slow Hand* by the Pointer sisters. We had been rehearsing it for months and our performance was flawless. I was wearing a red off the shoulder one piece pants suit and looked as glamorous as I felt. My father was in the audience along with thirty of my closest friends.

By this time, my father had been kicked out of the Mennonite Church for committing adultery and lying about it. I don't know if he had any judgement about my dancing, but if he did, he didn't say anything to me about it. Even though dancing was still considered a sin in the Mennonite Church, his "sins" had been so much greater than dancing, that he couldn't be judgmental about what I was doing. By the time of my 40th birthday, he and my mother had divorced and he was married to the woman he'd had an affair with. She and I weren't on friendly terms, and I hadn't invited her to the party.

Moving my body to music felt so natural and joyful—and it didn't lead to sex! I couldn't understand what had been sinful about it for all those years. Even if it hadn't been a sin to dance, I wonder if I could have enjoyed dancing when I was younger. I was so conditioned not to express myself, and dancing is another form of self-expression. Or the opposite could have happened. If I had been allowed to dance, I might have learned to express myself more.

This 40th birthday party was a demonstration of my freedom to express myself, without punishment. This was another opportunity to color outside the lines of the rules I had been raised to follow without question.

CHAPTER TWENTY-ONE
SPIRITUAL EVOLUTION

HASSAN WAS MY CHARMING IRANIAN Sunday School teacher while I was in graduate school at UCLA. I was gradually moving away from my rigid upbringing, but I was trying to find my place within a more liberal Christian Church. I attended a Presbyterian Church in LA that had an active college Sunday School class that I could get a ride to on Sundays. Hassan was also a student at UCLA, getting his PhD in linguistics. He lived near me, often gave me a ride, and we became friends. He was engaged to a woman named Carol, who I'd never met, but I thought of him as "safe" because he was engaged.

One Saturday when he was moving from one apartment to another, several of us from the Sunday School class helped him. At the end of the day, the others left because they had their own cars. I had to wait for him to take me home. He was tired, complaining of a backache, and I offered to give him a back rub, not understanding what that might mean in his culture. My sheltered Mennonite upbringing had not prepared me for the subtle and unexpected ways a sexual encounter could develop. I became less naïve that day, and I experienced another demonstration of what I labeled hypocrisy, or lack of integrity. My trust in Christians and the Christian church was being steadily eroded.

By the time I got my Masters in Social Work (MSW) degree from UCLA, I had gone to movies, tried drinking and smoking (didn't like either), was no longer a virgin, and was mostly free of the fear and rigidity of my Mennonite upbringing. It would be a few more years before I circled back around and discovered a rich and fulfilling spiritual life.

After graduate school I continued trying more liberal Christian churches, but I soon gave up on the need for a church. I couldn't find a community that aligned with my evolving beliefs. I missed the close community, but I developed a community of people I worked with and life became full without religion.

As my first husband and I got together, weekends were full with hiking and backpacking, then with clearing our land and building our house. And then Brian was born. When my husband started on the Scientology path, I took the Adventures in Attitudes training which was my first exposure to New Thought. I started reading books by Joseph Murphy and Catherine Ponder and found the Church of Religious Science (now called Center for Spiritual Living), and Unity. I hadn't realized how starved my soul was until it started to get fed.

I began attending church, taking classes, meditating, praying, and immersing myself in spiritual truths. I was introduced to the concept of the power of my thoughts and beliefs. I was introduced to affirmations, visualization, and the idea that my consciousness could create my reality.

After I became a single parent when Brian was two, I had an income that could barely pay for an apartment, but

I wanted to buy a house. I had been working ten hours a week for the County Mental Health Department and had a fixed and small income. Once Cathy and I started the Center for Health Awareness, my income would fluctuate, depending on how many seminars we organized and how many people signed up.

I immersed myself in prosperity consciousness, listening to audio tapes every day, doing affirmations, and visualizing. In four months, I quadrupled my income, enabling me to buy a house in an area with a great school district for Brian. This was a physical manifestation of the concepts I was learning, but the joy and meaning in life, as well as spiritual inner peace, was even more valuable.

Once we created the Center for Health Awareness, I started doing work that I loved—designing and teaching workshops on mind-body health for nurses. My seven years at the Center for Health Awareness, living in the house I bought, and raising Brian from ages three to ten, were some of the most stress-free, happy times of my life. I went to a body worker during that time who specialized in releasing trauma and negative emotions from the body. She told me after one session that there was nothing in my body for her to work on.

When the Center fell apart, causing a crisis of my faith, I lost the peace of my spiritual connection for a few years. It was during this spiritual desert that Brian went to live with his dad. I moved in with Michael and we started our furniture store business. Instead of getting spiritually fed on Sundays, I worked in the furniture store. Instead of reading spiritual texts and meditating, I worked twelve-hour days and fell into bed exhausted. Instead of spending time with friends and benefitting from social connections, I worked seven days a week.

A diagnosis of cancer woke me up. It brought me back to my center and to the importance of my spiritual connection. This is one of the gifts cancer gave me. I feel that my cancer diagnosis was an answer to my prayer, "Lord make me an instrument." I needed that wake-up call to get back on my true path and experience a meaningful purpose in life.

Spirituality and my connection to the Divine has been a driving force in enabling me to thrive with cancer for over thirty years. I believe in the omniscience and omnipresence of God, meaning that God is everywhere and everything. He/She isn't up in the sky judging us, but is the Energy that connects us, and all of Nature. A way of explaining this that resonates with me is that I have a finite self and an Infinite Self. My finite self is the individual called Jan who functions in daily life. My Infinite Self is the kingdom (or energy) of God that is within me. It is my spiritual Self. When the finite and the Infinite selves are connected, this is my super power. The Infinite me has all knowingness, is not afraid, and is at peace. The Infinite me isn't anxious waiting for test results. The Infinite me doesn't panic when cancer marker numbers go up.

The trick is not to let finite events eclipse the Infinite. I'm not saying this is easy to do. The world around us addresses only the finite self, and reminds us constantly of all the bad things that can happen and how much we need to be afraid. I have to consciously make an effort to stay in the peace of the Infinite Self. There are many tools that can help me—deep breathing, meditation, prayer, nature, laughter, music, quiet, meaning and purpose in life.

I believe the verse in the Bible (Romans 8:28) that says, "All things work together for good to those that love God." In practical terms, that means that anything that washes up on my beach (even cancer) is for my good. Things don't happen *to* me. They happen *for* me. I may not immediately see the goodness in an event or a diagnosis, but I know my finite viewpoint is limited. I trust that the goodness is there, and I look for it.

My spiritual life is an essential part of what has allowed me to live with cancer for over thirty years. Prayer, meditation, and daily reading of spiritual texts, along with a connection to a spiritual community, are all crucial components of keeping my spirit enlivened, my attitude optimistic, and my body healthy.

CHAPTER TWENTY-TWO

RUBY'S FUNERAL

RUBY WAS MY MOTHER'S SISTER, the one who'd locked me in a dark closet for hours when I was three for coloring outside the lines in my coloring book. Of course, I'd never warmed up to her after that. Ruby was the oldest of seven children, eighteen months older than my mother. My mother had been the first to die, and Ruby was second. When Aunt Ruby died, I decided to go to her funeral in Washington, not because I felt close to her, but because it was an opportunity to see the whole family together after such a long time.

I knew I would be risking another confrontation like I'd experienced when I was last with the family. The last time I saw the whole family, my mother's parents were still alive. My grandfather told me I was causing great distress and pain for the family because I was the only one in the extended family that wouldn't be in Heaven. They would all be together for eternity and were upset that I wasn't going to be with them. I alone would keep the whole family from being together forever. This was a family of missionaries and preachers who were immersed in the fundamental Christian world. Their belief was that I wasn't going to Heaven because I was no longer a born-again Christian, believing in the Lord Jesus Christ as my Savior. I was living a life of sin. I had lived with my husband before getting married. I no longer attended the Mennonite Church, or any other fundamental Christian church.

Even though I was hurt by my grandfather's incrimination of me, I also understood his position because I'd been there at one time. I'd thought that non-believers were going to Hell, and I wanted to help them find the truth. I knew my grandfather was in pain because I was coloring outside his lines.

I decided then that I didn't need to visit them again since it brought pain to both of us. They lived in Oregon and I lived in California. They died a few years after that incident, and I never saw them again. I also didn't see the rest of the family although I have stayed in touch with my mother's youngest two sisters who are still alive. Aunt Jane and Aunt Susan consistently send me birthday cards and/ or call me on my birthday. We often say "I love you" to each other, and our love for each other is genuine. Because I know what their beliefs are about my soul going to Hell, I know they are praying for me and hoping I will come back to the fold. I'm grateful they didn't talk to me about it when we were together for Ruby's funeral and that we could focus on the love we have for each other instead of our differences.

The only other family member who had directly confronted me with my "sinful" ways was Uncle Leo, my mother's oldest brother. He'd written me a letter once to tell me that my work with Healing Journeys was "of the Devil." He said the only way anyone's life could be improved was for them to accept Jesus as their personal

Savior. Any other help offered to people was misleading, a lie, and of the Devil. I never responded to Uncle Leo's letter, and I dreaded being confronted by him in person.

I knew all five remaining siblings, spouses, kids, and grandkids would be at Aunt Ruby's funeral which would be held in Lyndon, Washington, where Aunt Susan, the youngest sister, still lived. The other two remaining sisters would be staying at Susan's house, and I was invited to stay there too as the representative of their older sister.

I had many warm and positive memories of family gatherings as a child and I wanted to see some of my relatives, especially Jane who became my favorite aunt when she lived with us as a teenager. She was eleven years older than I was and we shared a room in our house when she was in her last year of high school. Since my mother was sickly, and I felt I had to prepare for her death, Jane had agreed that I could live with her if Mom died while I was still a child.

With the whole family together for Ruby's funeral, I thought as long as I could avoid individual contact with Uncle Leo, I could dodge the discomfort of a confrontation. Once we were all together, it didn't take me long to realize that Uncle Leo was on his way to dementia and we wouldn't be having a meaningful conversation. I was relieved. None of the other aunts, uncles or cousins had ever confronted me directly so I relaxed and enjoyed sharing memories and stories and laughing together.

On the last day there, my cousin Wes asked if we could go outside and have a private conversation. I was the oldest grandchild and Wes was the next oldest, the cousin closest to my age. He lived in Bakersfield, CA, and was Ruby's only living son. I thought, "Oh no, here it comes. I never expected to get it from Wes."

Once outside, his opening question was, "What is your current belief about God?" I responded that I believed God was everywhere and everything, but I no longer believed what we were taught growing up. I no longer believed there was a Heaven and Hell where we would spend eternity, depending on whether we believed in Jesus as the only son of God who died for our sins. I said my understanding of God had expanded to a more loving and inclusive God.

Wes was my friend on Facebook and had been watching my posts for several years. He had suspected I no longer held our Mennonite values, and he said he thought maybe I was right. Even though he was questioning, he had continued going to the Mennonite church as long as his mother was alive and he was taking her to church. He didn't want to upset her by questioning her values. He said he had heard how the sisters had berated me, and he didn't want to experience their judgement. Now that she was gone, he and his wife were going to explore other options.

I was shocked. I had never had such a conversation with anyone in the family. I finally felt like someone in the family saw the real me and didn't feel compelled to change me. I had an ally in the family who accepted me as I was. I felt grateful and a little less alone.

CHAPTER TWENTY-THREE

SYMPATHY SHAVE

I'VE BEEN TOLD THAT WHEN I was born with red hair, my mother cried. There were no redheads in our family, in either my grandparents' or parents' generations. But, my mother's grandfather had a red beard, so my mother knew there was a remote possibility that she could birth a redhead. To her, red hair was almost like a curse, and she couldn't see anyone with red hair as attractive.

My mother took my red hair seriously by limiting what I could wear. She thought red, pink, or orange didn't go with red hair so those colors were off-limits. My older cousin used to give me hand-me-down clothes. In grade school she gave me a beautiful hot pink dress that I loved, but my mother never let me wear it because in her eyes, it "clashed" with my hair.

Sometimes, as a child, people stopped me on the street to ask where I got my beautiful red hair, but in spite of these compliments, I still thought my red hair was undesirable until junior high school when I met Sue Henryson, possibly the most popular girl in school, who had flaming red hair. She was the head cheerleader, and later won the Miss California pageant. Clearly red hair hadn't held her back. After that, in junior high school, my friend Diane told me she envied my red hair. She had "mousy" brown hair and said she never stood out in a crowd like I did. I learned to love being a redhead.

When the color began fading in my fifties, I started dying my hair to keep it red. I was married to a man eleven years my junior and had occasionally been mistaken for his mother. I wanted to look as young as possible to keep that from happening again, but I started wondering what all those chemicals were doing to my body. And I thought about how much money I'd save by not dying my hair every five weeks. But how does one go from red to whatever is underneath without an awkward two-tone phase?

When my friend Patty was losing her hair as a result of chemo for her lymphoma, I had an answer. A "sympathy shave." I could be bald in sympathy for Patty's baldness. Patty agreed to shave my head. On October 31, 2009, we made a ritual out of it, and also had some fun with it. Patty's hair loss process was just starting and she had shaved everything except a tall Mohawk down the middle, dyed in bright colors. She shaved mine in the same design. I still have some great pictures of us in this in-between Mohawk stage. We had the whole head-shaving process videotaped, including my tears as she made the first pass and I saw my beautiful red hair in a heap on the floor.

People had often called me courageous, but I hadn't felt courageous when I was responding to something I had no choice in, and simply had to handle what was in front of me. This was different. This was my decision and was the first time I truly felt courageous. I didn't know what would be left when all the red was gone. Who would I be when I no longer stood out in a crowd because I was a redhead? I felt the grief of giving up a part of my identity.

I hadn't anticipated a positive reaction to having a bald head! When I went to church bald, people wanted to feel my head. At first, they thought I had lost my hair because of my own cancer and chemo, but when they found out I did it as a sympathy shave for Patty, they were impressed. I felt sexy with a bald head. Strangers stopped me on the street to tell me my head was beautifully shaped. As my own hair came in white, I called it platinum blonde, and was pleased with the number of positive comments my new hair elicited.

I still stand out in a crowd because my hair is a vibrant white. When I'm standing in the sun, people have said my hair looks like a halo. If someone asked me where I got my white hair, I would have to give the same answer I did when people questioned where I got my red hair. "God gave it to me," and I'm grateful.

If being copied is the sincerest complement, I got that, too. Within a few months, at least five other women at church had quit dying their hair, telling me they were inspired by my example.

CHAPTER TWENTY-FOUR

BELONGING TO SOMETHING LARGER

All things work together for good to those that love God.
~ Romans 8:28

MY FRIEND, LINDSAY, TEXTED TO tell me Tara Brach (a prominent meditation teacher) had quoted me in her podcast. Wow! I was curious. I had attended a workshop with Tara Brach many years before, but she didn't know me. Eager to find out what I had said that was worth quoting, I listened to the podcast, entitled, "Shifting from Limbic to Liberating Intention." Tara talked about how important it is to know what really matters in our lives and what our deepest intentions are. She said in our day-to-day lives, we often lose track of our deepest intentions and get caught up with intentions that don't matter at the deepest level. For example, we may cut someone off in traffic to try to get somewhere on time, forgetting that our deepest intention is to be kind. Or, we may be stubborn in an argument with a friend, trying to be right, forgetting that our deepest intention is connection.

This is the story I wrote in a Healing Journeys eNews-letter in 2010 that Tara shared in this podcast....

Following my ocular melanoma in 2007, I had an annual chest X-ray to see if melanoma had metastasized to my lungs. After my chest X-ray in 2010, I had a call from my doctor the very next day and knew this wouldn't be good news. There was a nodule on my lung and he wanted me to have a CT scan. I got the scan done on a Wednesday and the technician said my doctor would have the results the next morning.

I was oddly impressed with how quickly my anxiety level went over the top. On Thursday I couldn't concentrate and I felt like crying all day. I kept thinking about what I would do if I found out I had metastatic cancer. Would it mean that all the diet, exercise, and lifestyle strategies I was using hadn't made a difference? I might as well go back to enjoying Root Beer Floats. I felt angry and disappointed, and I didn't have the energy left to fight cancer anymore. I called my doctor's office twice and was promised he would call me before the end of the day. He didn't.

Something happened Thursday night as I read and meditated. I remembered my prayer to "make me an instrument" and to "use me." What if my having metastatic cancer was the way I could be most useful—as an inspiration to others somehow?

It's more important to me that my life be meaningful rather than easy. I don't want to judge any experience as bad or good, but accept whatever washes up on my beach as part of the package. I believe that "all things work together for good." That was on a plaque in my parents' home as I was growing up and it has always brought me comfort. Thinking about that, I became peaceful and calm, and I had a restful night's sleep.

On Friday I called my doctor's office again and was told he had left for a two-week vacation. How could he have abandoned me like that? I asked if they had the results of my CT scan and they did. I asked to please have the on-call doctor call me and give me the results. By six p.m. I hadn't received a phone call and was surprised that I was hardly thinking about it anymore. I was feeling okay with whatever would be. No more anxiety. I could have a good weekend without knowing the results.

At 8:30 p.m. I noticed there was a message on my cell phone. My phone had been with me all day. I hadn't heard it ring and hadn't seen the message notification from the on-call doctor. She said she'd compared my CT scan with a 2007 scan. The nodule had been there in 2007 and it hadn't changed. She said it was nothing to worry about because it was stable. I didn't even know it had been detected previously. Maybe all my efforts were having an impact. Hurray! I emailed all my friends who had been praying for me, and I celebrated. Even though I was OK with whatever happened, it was, of course, still my preference that cancer didn't progress.

In retrospect, I'm glad I didn't get the results right away. The extra time gave me the opportunity to get in touch with my inner strength and my inner knowing that I would be okay no matter what. I'm not just a body. Someday I know this body won't go on, and I will still be okay. I like being reminded of that periodically.

Tara used this story as an example of how I'd gotten in touch with my deepest intention, which is to be an instrument. My intention is that my life serve something larger than myself. Tara also spoke about the way this created a sense of belonging for me. She believed that belonging to something larger than ourselves is what carries us through this living-dying world. Whatever happens in my life is an essential part of this larger world to which I belong.

I think this is the key to my being mostly calm and accepting during my years of living with cancer. I know that whatever happens in my life is necessary for manifesting the fullness of who I have come here to be. From my limited human perspective, I can't understand the "bad" things that happen to me, but I trust that my life experiences will support and enhance my deepest intention to be an instrument. I have a quote taped to my desk that says, "The purpose of our aliveness is to strike our gift against the needs of the world." As long as I'm alive, that's what I want to do.

CHAPTER TWENTY-FIVE

SYNCHRONICITY

I AM SITTING IN THE waiting area of the restaurant of the Marriott in Santa Clara, California, regrouping and trying to think of a Plan B. I had hoped to talk to Lawrence LeShan when his workshop finished, but I just missed him. I want to meet Dr. LeShan and acquire permission to use the title of his book, "Cancer as a Turning Point," for the program I'm designing for anyone touched by cancer.

I'd been living in San Jose, California, and had seen an ad for his pre-conference workshop nearby, at the Marriott in Santa Clara. I was already planning to attend the weekend conference, but I had to work the day of his workshop. I'd hoped I could show up by the end of his workshop and get a chance to talk to him, but I hadn't counted on the heavy traffic and he was gone by the time I got to his workshop room. He wasn't scheduled to speak at the weekend conference.

I decided to have dinner in the restaurant at the Marriott while I figured out a Plan B. There was a line, so I was seated in the waiting area. A couple sat next to me, also waiting for dinner. He looked familiar—I had seen Lawrence LeShan's picture. What are the chances that, in this crowded hotel, he would sit right next to me? I've learned that when I am doing what gives me life, the

Universe supports me, and the chances of this happening are abundant. This knowledge gave me the courage to ask if he was Lawrence LeShan. Of course, it was Larry.

We had a ten-minute conversation that day that ended with him saying, "You have not only my permission, but also my blessings." Years later, when he attended one of the conferences as a speaker, he told me how happy he was that someone was making use of his work and carrying it forward. As I am writing this, I'm remembering that Larry had just celebrated his 100th birthday. On November 10, 2020, two months following his 100th birthday, Larry passed. I'm happy to have called this amazing and generous man my friend.

The synchronicity of that meeting was the encouragement I needed to move forward with producing the conference. The first one was in 1994 in a hotel on the beach in Monterey, California. It was advertised as a conference for women; all the presenters were women, and there were 280 women in the audience. The presenters included well-known women who had authored books, like Jean Shinoda Bolen, MD, and Jeanne Achterberg, PhD. Also included was a humorist, a singer, a Taiko drum group, and healing stories from women who were thriving while dealing with cancer.

Our mission at Healing Journeys was to support healing, activate hope, and promote thriving. Our focus was on healing rather than curing. We differentiated between them based on the work of Carol Ritberger, PhD, as follows:

HEALING	CURING
Is done by you	Is done to you
Happens from the inside out	Happens from the outside in
Is active	Is passive
Addresses the cause	Addresses the symptom
Encompasses all of you	Singles out one part of you
Is gradual but long-lasting	Is quick but short-lived
Leaves you better than you were before	Restores you to where you were
Focuses on you	Focuses on the ailment

The conference wasn't about medical treatments, but about what we could do for ourselves to stimulate our self-healing abilities. My criteria in selecting presenters included authenticity and an ability to connect with the audience. We always included music and humor, languages of the soul. We started every conference with a local singer singing the *Hero Song* by Mariah Carey. I introduced it by asking people to imagine that the singer was singing these words just to them.

The lyrics of the song ask people to look inside their hearts, reach into their souls, and find their strength within. When we feel like hope is gone, we can look inside for courage. The truth is that a hero lies inside each one of us (you can hear Mariah Carey sing *Hero* at https://www.youtube.com/watch?v=0IA3ZvCkRkQ).

There were often not many dry eyes at the end of that song. People took in the message and their hearts were opened. That first weekend conference was everything I had hoped it would be and more. People left feeling inspired, hopeful, and full. I used the metaphor that the conference was like a buffet. They had consumed so much that they felt like they may never need to eat again. But they would get hungry again. I asked them to pay attention to what fed their spirit over the two days of the conference, so they would know what they needed next time their spirit was hungry.

Some people were fed by listening to speakers. We recorded the presenters and they could easily take home tapes or CDs and listen to them again. Some people said the most meaningful experience for them was making deep connections with others in similar situations. Long-term support groups were formed and continued after the conference. Some people told me they learned how much music affected how they felt, and they listened to music more consciously after the conference. For others it was humor they needed more of. For many, it was knowing they weren't alone, and that knowledge stayed with them. We wanted to nurture people at the deepest level and I was delighted when someone called the conference "A Broadway Show for the Soul."

CHAPTER TWENTY-SIX

A BROADWAY SHOW FOR THE SOUL

I'M VOLUNTEERING AT SOMEONE ELSE'S conference in San Francisco in order to receive a discount on the fee so I can attend. I'm a door monitor, watching for name badges as people enter the auditorium. A woman I don't recognize walks through the door and asks me, "Are you the lady who did the cancer conference?" When I say yes, she throws her arms around me and, sobbing in my arms, says "You saved my life. When I was diagnosed with cancer, I thought it was a death sentence and I was hunkered down at home, dying. A friend took me, kicking and screaming, to your conference. By the end of the two days, I knew cancer could be a life sentence, and I'm now thriving."

This is just one example of the feedback I received after that first magical *Cancer as a Turning Point, From Surviving to Thriving*™ weekend conference on the beach in Monterey. I heard from so many people how inspiring and empowering it was that I felt compelled to do it again. And again. The evolution of the conferences was fed by the reactions of the attendees and slowly unfolded with a magnetic energy that attracted not only more and more cancer patients, but incredible volunteers who seemed to emerge from everywhere. Those first two years, I produced conferences in San Diego, San Francisco, Huntington

Beach, and Sacramento. I promoted them as conferences for women and all the presenters were women. I insisted they happen in hotels on the beach because of the feminine, healing influence of water.

The one in Sacramento was a challenge. Fran Haynes, who later became a Healing Journeys Board member, had attended the first conference in Monterey. She hadn't been diagnosed with cancer, but she'd had a cancer scare. She had micro calcifications in her breast and was afraid they would turn into cancer. She felt so emotionally and spiritually fed at that first conference that she wanted it to happen in Sacramento closer to her home. Sacramento is not on the beach. When she called to request a Sacramento conference, I told her if she could find a hotel in Sacramento that was next to water, I would consider it. She found the Radisson Hotel which has a man-made lake in the center of it. Even though it was trapped water, it was still water.

At that time, we charged $195 for these weekend conferences, and gave scholarships to anyone who asked. The attendance ranged from 90 to 280. The feedback I received from participants continued to pour in and was so powerful that we had to continue. This was feeling like my "assignment." It was definitely an answer to my prayer to "make me an instrument." Producing this conference used many of the skills I had developed in other jobs over the years, and was a powerful way to utilize my gifts to benefit others. It was also beneficial for me on my own healing journey. As I went to other conferences and read books in the search for presenters for my program, I was acquiring tools to support my own healing as well as benefitting hundreds of others.

But the conferences weren't yet a way for me to make a living. The furniture store business that Michael and I had created was paying the bills. Healing Journeys was more of a hobby, but an expensive hobby. After two years and five conferences, I was personally $35,000 in debt. The income couldn't cover the expenses.

Then, amazingly, I received an unsolicited check in the mail for $5,000 from a woman who had attended the conference in San Francisco and wanted them to continue. Since I had formed Healing Journeys as a non-profit organization, donations could be tax-deductible. This unexpected contribution helped birth the counter-intuitive idea to offer the conference free and ask for donations.

This donation was one of several large unsolicited donations that would arrive through the years. Often, just when I was exhausted from fund-raising and thinking I couldn't do it anymore, an unexpected contribution would arrive. One year we received a check for $60,000 from the estate of Toni Minvielle. I didn't know Toni, but she had attended our conference in Oakland in 1998 and because the conference made such a difference in her life, she wanted to ensure we could continue. Toni had donated her IRA to Healing Journeys when she died. She wanted to contribute to a small organization where her support would make a difference, and it did! I thought of Toni often, and was motivated to keep going because of her belief in us.

For our first free conference, I was also able to persuade a non-profit organization associated with Stanford University to co-sponsor the conference on the Stanford campus and secure an auditorium at no charge. Attendance at our first free conference at Stanford in 1996 jumped from the 90 to 280 range to 1400! Our strategy, that felt so in alignment with the needs of cancer patients and their caregivers, was working! Now, the fee couldn't prevent anyone from attending.

I had reached out to speakers I thought would bring cutting-edge information, joy and inspiration to the audience. Some were well-known authors like Rachel Naomi Remen, MD; Jean Shinoda Bolen, MD; Dawna Markova, PhD; and Marion Woodman, Jungian Analyst; who each said yes to being part of this new kind of conference that would bring women together in a safe, healing space. Other signature components of every conference were music, humor, drama, dance, drumming, a speaker on nutrition, healing stories, and lunch networking groups.

My job as emcee for the event was much bigger than simply introducing speakers. In the new-age vernacular, I was "holding the space." I'd attended conferences where the conference organizer introduced a speaker and then left the auditorium, presumably to do more important work. My philosophy was that there was *nothing more important than what was happening on stage*. I sat in the front row as a good listener for every presenter. I was communicating my belief in the importance of what was being presented. And I was making the space emotionally safe, creating a "container" for the presentations to be most effective. The audience learned that I vetted each speaker, and that I was monitoring what was being presented. They could relax and take everything in because they trusted me.

The onstage programs were educational and inspirational, but much of the value of the event came from the community. On the evaluation forms, we asked what was most valuable to participants. One woman responded "the bathroom line." While standing in line, she'd overheard a conversation between two other women. One of them said she'd had twenty-six lymph nodes involved when she had her mastectomy a number of years before. The woman overhearing this had just had surgery in which twelve lymph nodes were cancerous and she'd thought that was a death sentence. Hearing that someone else had survived a much more dire circumstance gave her hope.

Some people said the lunch networking groups were the most valuable part of the conference. We placed signs on the tables that called out different kinds of cancer so people who wanted to meet someone with the same kind of cancer could have that opportunity. Volunteers helped the women find each other. Some people with rare cancers had never before met anyone with the same cancer. The two women with leiomyosarcoma (a malignant [cancerous] smooth muscle tumor affecting one in 100,000 people) became long-lasting friends. Support groups were formed that continued for years. The women with double mastectomies shared their experiences and their scars with each other. People using complementary treatments were able to share what they had tried and what had or hadn't worked for them. Breast cancer survivors with young children were able to share strategies for talking to their children about their disease.

Most of these lunch networking groups had deep and

meaningful conversations. One exception might be the men (who were now being included) with prostate cancer. I heard from one of them that they were more comfortable talking about sports than their experience of cancer. But who am I to say that wasn't a useful connection for them? Just knowing they weren't alone in their cancer experience could have been beneficial.

We also used the lunch time to practice what we preached about nutrition. Our snacks and lunches were organic and we tried to keep them low-carb and full of fresh vegetables and fruits. No sugar. Although the conference was free, people pre-ordered and paid for their lunches. We charged only what it cost us for the lunch without any profit.

With the attendance going from an average of 150 to 1400 by making the conference free, the Healing Journeys board committed that we would always offer the conference at no charge. The Stanford conference was the first one to pay for itself because the Stanford facility was provided, most of the speakers waived their fees, I wasn't being compensated, and we received donations from attendees. The donations covered the costs of marketing, equipment rental, a sound technician, office assistance for preparations, and office costs.

However, a business model of finding free venues and not paying speakers or staff wasn't sustainable. A big part of my job became fundraising—writing grant proposals, getting sponsors for the conference, and asking people for contributions. One of the grantors required that the conference not be promoted as a women-only conference, but be promoted to both men and women, and include male presenters. This felt like the next step in our growth and the Board agreed. The conference grew into a profound experience for anyone touched by cancer or any life-altering condition. One participant said it was for anyone with a heart.

Our typical audience was 50 percent cancer survivors, 25 percent support people, 20 percent health professionals (we offered continuing education credits to nurses and counselors), and 5 percent volunteers and speakers. My interest and expertise lay in what happened on stage, but much of the "work" of the conference happened elsewhere. We often had up to fifty volunteers assisting with all the aspects of producing the event. I'm grateful to Carol Purin, our first Healing Journeys Board president, and part-time employee, for organizing the volunteer jobs and the people doing them. Carol was a three-time survivor of Lymphoma, and a retired nursing instructor. She had seen cancer from both sides, had utilized both Western medicine and alternative treatments, and her heart resonated with the mission of the conference to support healing, activate hope, and promote thriving.

It was challenging to register a thousand-plus people in less than an hour, serve snacks and coffee in a thirty-minute break, set up and monitor a comfort room for those who needed to rest, supervise child care, maintain lost and found, organize lunch networking groups, serve lunch, and staff an information table in the lobby to deal with every need that came up. With fifty volunteers, there had to be team leaders, and everyone had to be trained. Carol created binders with job descriptions for every job, trained people ahead of time, and helped create an atmosphere of loving kindness. In training volunteers, Carol always said "these people may look normal, but they're all going through something hard and need kindness."

And then there were the Sugar Plump Fairies, founded and organized by Fran Haynes, currently the longest serving Healing Journeys board member. Fran had attended Wavy Gravy's Clown Camp every summer and was a master at lightening up the atmosphere. Most of the Fairies (including Fran) were therapists on their day jobs. At the conference they greeted people as they arrived at the entrance sites. They dressed outrageously, exaggerating a high school prom vibe with blue hair, wildly extreme hats and boas, long flashy gowns finished off with tennis shoes, and, oh yes, bubbles! They moved through the crowd laughing, welcoming attendees by blowing bubbles in, around and over their heads, giving off a festive, hopeful vibe. They brought extra hats and boas for those participants inclined to join them in their vibrant, uplifting spirit for the weekend, and many took advantage of the offer. Joy and laughter wasn't what people touched by a life-threatening illness expected at a cancer conference, and when they saw all that joy, some thought at first that they must be in the wrong place.

We also had a professional photographer taking pictures of participants as they arrived, often interacting with a Sugar Plump Fairy. The photographer created a slide show which we showed at the closing of each conference. We called it a "Celebration of Heroes" and the images were accompanied with John Denver's uplifting, comforting rendition of "All This Joy."

Feeling that joy may have been the first step toward seeing cancer as a transformational experience rather than a death sentence. For many people, the conference was a turning point in their attitude toward their cancer and their healing journey. They left feeling inspired and hopeful, connected and not alone, and with many resources to access as they continued their healing journeys.

~

CHAPTER TWENTY-SEVEN

HOW DID WE GET TO GREENVILLE?

ROSEMARY COULD FEEL THE ENERGY course through her body as she pounded the big drums on stage at the *Cancer as a Turning Point*™ conference at UC Davis in 2001. Rosemary, a breast cancer survivor, was about five-feet tall, but felt big and strong as she beat the huge Taiko drums. At the end of their performance, the Taiko group had invited anyone from the audience who wanted to experience beating the drums to come up on stage. This was such an empowering experience for Rosemary that she went home to Seattle and asked the American Cancer Society (ACS) to help bring the conference to Seattle. Rosemary was a "Reach to Recovery" volunteer for ACS in Seattle. Her experience of beating the big drums on stage with the Taiko drum group had been so profound for her that she wanted to share the experience with the women she supported through ACS.

The first I knew of this was when Debra from Seattle ACS called me and asked if we would bring our conference to Seattle. Our estimated budget for a two-day conference at that time was about $100,000. She said ACS would cover $25,000 of the costs if I could raise the rest of the money. I went to work.

Fortunately, my son was living in Seattle at the time

and I got to see him about once a month for a year as I went to Seattle for planning meetings. I found the perfect venue in Meany Hall at the University of Washington. Lynne Singer, one of the Healing Journeys board members, had just moved to Seattle and had helped create a steering committee of local residents to help with the planning.

We collaborated with a local non-profit, Cancer Lifeline. The director at the time, Barbara Frederick, had been best friends with Mary Gates, Bill Gates' mother. Barbara had continued the friendship with Bill and Melinda. Barbara arranged a meeting with a representative from the Gates Foundation and, to my delight, they contributed $20,000, on the condition that we wouldn't ask again. They believed strongly that the local community should take over funding resources after this initial offering of support.

There are many cancer centers in the Seattle area and I met with each one of them to solicit sponsorship. Most of them contributed, but many at minimal levels ($1,000). The first of three Seattle conferences happened in 2003. The Sugar Plump Fairies, Healing Journeys board members, and many California volunteers traveled to Seattle at their own expense to make it happen successfully.

It was at a Seattle conference that the seed of a Greenville, South Carolina, conference was watered. The seed had been planted by the CD sets of talks from previous conferences, recorded and marketed by Sounds True. Robin, a cancer patient in Greenville, bought the CD set at Barnes and Noble. After listening to them, Robin called me and asked what it would take to bring the conference to Greenville, South Carolina.

I told Robin that it would take someone passionate to do the local organizing. I said, "If you're serious about this, you need to come to a conference. Only an actual conference experience will give you the level of passion required to carry through with the project."

Robin and her husband, Denby, flew to Seattle and attended the conference. Denby, a prominent lawyer in Greenville, went along to placate his wife. He took a book with him and planned to sit in the audience reading while Robin checked out the conference. Robin said it didn't take long for Denby to put his book away and become totally engaged in the experience. What really got his attention was Annan Paterson's one-woman drama, *Deep Canyon*. When referring to hospital food, she said, "How do they fuck up jello?" Robin and Denby were both on board.

I had never heard of Greenville and had no desire to go to South Carolina, but because Healing Journeys felt like my "assignment," I was open to what I perceived as Spirit's direction. Robin created a steering committee in Greenville, consisting of her oncologist, and some of the movers and shakers in the community. I agreed to go meet with them.

I almost felt like I was in another country when I first met with the Greenville steering committee. They all "talked funny" with their Southern accents, insisted on calling me Ma'am, and expected someone from California to be a little weird. They weren't familiar with the speakers that were so well known in California, and needed me to justify many of my decisions about the event. Why do the lunches have to be organic? Why include music and humor in the conference? Fortunately, because of Robin's long-standing respect and admiration in the community, they were open and eager to absorb new information. Robin told me later she thought our conference had changed cancer care in Greenville. I would say that Robin changed cancer care in Greenville. She was the driving force. I almost felt like I had cloned myself in Robin, who wanted to establish and be in charge of an East Coast division of Healing Journeys and bring the conference to many cities. Robin was one of the most passionate, dedicated, generous, open, proactive, loving people I have ever met. We became sisters of the heart and I can now say one of the gifts I received from cancer was getting to know Robin, and all the precious people in Greenville, South Carolina.

From 2005 to 2009, we produced three conferences in Greenville. After Robin's cancer progressed, she died in January, 2008. As a result of the work she had started, following her death, we were able to produce conferences in Spartanburg, South Carolina; Charlottesville, Virginia; and Knoxville, Tennessee. Our workshop, *The Cancer-Fighting Kitchen,* was offered in Greer, South Carolina, and Macon, Georgia. These life-changing events happened because both Robin and I had cancer and were dedicated to using what we were learning to benefit others.

From 1994 to 2018, Healing Journeys produced thirty-seven *Cancer as a Turning Point*™ conferences in six states. More than 25,000 people attended. It became hard to count how many unique attendees there were because there were so many repeaters. People came back for the inspiration, the spiritual nurturing, and to bring family and friends with them.

There was a group of five or six brain cancer patients from Sacramento who, for several years, traveled together to wherever our conference was, to celebrate life, to be inspired again, and to connect with and support each other. The mother of one of the patients organized the group and accompanied them. Several of them told their stories at a conference and the inspiration went both ways.

Many times, after a conference, a participant would ask me why I didn't tell them ahead of time how powerful it would be. They would have brought everyone they knew with them. I wasn't able to find words that could adequately convey the depth of experience the audience had. Maybe you can get a sense of the experience by reading a participant's point of view. Following one of our Greenville conferences, a participant, Amy Webb, sent me the following essay she had written about her experience:

The Conference That Turned Us

The week after my lumpectomy I received in the mail a brochure inviting me to a free conference entitled, *Cancer as a Turning Point...From Surviving to Thriving*. As I read through the information, the more intrigued and pulled I felt. The crystal ball was mute for four months hence, but I registered the next day, keeping the brochure on my desk, in plain sight.

The timing was a bit off — I'd be between my fifth and last chemo treatment, but it was only a five-hour drive, on my 20th wedding anniversary weekend, and I imagined it as a possible celebration. My husband Richard readily agreed to accompany me, checking off the space on the registration form, "Family Caregiver/Support."

As months of treatment progressed, and my white counts took the quick elevator to the basement, the oncologist urged me to stay out of germs' way, avoiding crowds and sick people. For weeks I chose to go to the sparsely attended first service at church, if I felt up to that, and generally cocooned myself. This paid off, as I had to deal only with chemo aftereffects, and nothing else physically taxing during those months.

The appointment for blood count analysis after my fifth treatment was the day before we'd have to leave for the conference. I made my husband a deal—if the counts were up, we'd go. They were—miraculously against the trend. I called him from the parking lot outside the oncologist's office and rejoiced, "Pack your bags!" This would be my first time away in six months, a far cry from the nearly two decades of almost weekly travel that had previously been a part of my job.

Furman University's campus proved to be a sanctuary. Cars filled the parking lot, although the school year had ended. The walkways to the auditorium were filled with what looked like couples of all ages, women with sisters or friends, solo acts. I looked around for those in hats, but most had hair, and I immediately felt a bit self-conscious.

Although I needed my hat for cover in the sun, it was too hot for wearing very long in the southern summer. I worried my baldness would stand out, revealing me as in-treatment, still underway. I comforted myself by remembering a friend's compliment about sporting a great shaped head. And I purposely wore great outrageous earrings that belonged in the Caribbean.

The auditorium was fairly dark, despite the bright morning. Almost every seat was filled. It was quiet as a cathedral, except for the flutist on stage improvising medleys. As I heard her breathe, I could take a deep breath. I could feel myself intensely curious, feeling for the first time that my cancer diagnosis was a ticket into something huge.

We sat toward the back; the inclined floor allowed us to see a grand sweep of stage and flock. The lights went on and the program began. Singers, speakers, authors, composers, doctors, nutritionists, dancers, musicians, and story-tellers gifted us with their wisdom, energy, and admission of how their lives had been transformed by the very disease that brought us all together.

The pace worked, energizing as it flowed. Soon into the two days, I put away my notebook and simply absorbed the program. My husband and I stood side-by-side in guided yoga stretches. We sat moved by more than one performer's movement to music that unfolded a picture of a treacherous path and graceful passage. We sang. We laughed. We listened—a liturgy, gentle and strong—professed surviving as opportunity, fully recognizing that not all before us would be easy.

I thought now and then about what I would share in my summary emails to my circle of support, so many images opening me like a kaleidoscope. It seemed impossible to do justice to this experience by putting it into words. The essence of community was more powerful than craft.

What to include? What to leave out? Certainly, I needed to spotlight the opening request from Jan for survivors and then caregivers to stand. To hear all of us applauding each other in a wordless L'Chaim! was profoundly moving. Harder, though, for readers to see through my tears that final digital montage of candid photos, presented as, *Celebrating Heroes*.

As we stood to leave the auditorium, music blaring, I called over our seats to one amazing actress as she was walking out before us. Jonna had staged a one-woman masterpiece, depicting her own several rounds of cancer and treatments, a portrayal which made me howl with laughter, nod in knowing, wince, and sob.

"Thank you, thank you for showing me what can come on the other side," I had said to her. "You are a gift to the world." She hugged me close, her full head of curly hair brushing my baldness. And we both cried. Then she crouched down beside Richard, willing to wait for me to snap a picture of them together. I noticed that as I was putting my camera away, she spoke briefly to him.

On the walk back to the car, my husband asked me what I said to her. The report choked in my throat and instead of answering him, I asked him what she'd said to him in parting.

"She told me she had been sitting a couple rows behind us during some of the performances, watching me rub your head. She said how much it touched her, how moving to see so much love," he replied.

We both went silent. Then he added, "I heard her words and thought, 'I did this? I had this impact? I was merely doing what felt good to me.'"

That not-so-long drive home was filled with silent memorializing and plenty of conversation. We were not the same couple we had been just three days ago. We wondered aloud what the other side would look like for us, how emergence would translate. Without saying another word, we signed on to find out.

~

Strategies
for Managing
Cancer

CHAPTER TWENTY-EIGHT

NUTRITION

Eat food. Not too much. Mostly plants.
~ Michael Pollan

WHEN I COUNSEL NEWLY DIAGNOSED cancer patients, often their first question is the same as mine was in 1989 – "what shall I eat?" Although there are still some doctors who tell a patient to eat whatever she wants because it doesn't matter, most health professionals now know that what we eat matters a great deal.

When I was sixteen, as you read in Chapter Three, "Undiagnosed Illness," I learned that what I put in my mouth matters. So, the first expert I looked for after being diagnosed with cancer was a nutritionist. My first nutritionist had worked for Cancer Treatment Centers of America, and had written a book on cancer and nutrition (currently out of print). She recommended a low-fat vegetarian diet for me, as did most "experts" at that time. She didn't tell me to avoid processed foods, but recommended that less than 30 percent of my calories come from fat. I meticulously read labels, looking at the fat content, but not necessarily at the sugar content. I didn't realize then that when they took out fat, sugar was added to make the food more flavorful. We now know that sugar feeds cancer more than fat does.

I stayed on that vegetarian diet for twelve years, but eventually started questioning the low-fat part. People were starting to talk about the importance of eating whole foods, and low fat yogurt isn't a whole food. It's altered by taking the fat out of it.

During the years I lived in Santa Cruz (1995 to 2002), I met Jeanne Wallace, PhD, who was studying nutrition. She became interested in nutrition and cancer when her partner was diagnosed with a glioblastoma (brain cancer). Jeanne would give lectures to small groups of people locally and could easily talk for three hours about the research on beating cancer with nutrition. I was fascinated with the depth of her knowledge and never got tired of learning from her. Because of Jeanne's nutritional "treatment," her partner, who had a two percent chance of survival, is still alive and well as of this writing.

After Jeanne got her PhD in nutrition, she was my nutritionist for many years. She steeped herself in the latest research, and ordered blood tests to individualize recommendations to my body's needs. Jeanne's knowledge is so deep and comprehensive that I asked her why she didn't write a book. She said the research changes our knowledge so often that a book would be out of date by the time it was published.

During the twelve years I was a vegetarian, I had almost annual local recurrences of cancer under my left arm. Then in 2002, I had not only a recurrence under my left arm, but also a new cancer in my right breast. This felt like a sign that something needed to change.

That's when I read Dr. Harold Kristal's book, *The Nutrition Solution: A Guide to Your Metabolic Type*. Your metabolic type is the fundamental way in which your body produces and processes energy. Different people need different kinds of foods; one person's nourishment is another's poison. The trick is to discover what kinds of foods your individual metabolism thrives on. That's where metabolic testing came in.

I was tested for my metabolic type and was told I needed to be eating meat, ideally at every meal. In 2002, I started eating meat, but was selective in the quality of the meat. I learned that the research that claimed meat was carcinogenic was based on eating meat from Concentrated Animal Feeding Operations (CAFO). These animals are fed a diet that is not natural to them and, as a result, these animals are not well. The same research based on meat from animals that are fed their natural diet (grass-fed and grass-finished beef) revealed that meat was cancer protective. I also remembered that the diet Dr. Friesen recommended when I was sixteen included abundant red meat. If it contributed to my healing then, maybe it would be beneficial now. I started eating chicken that was free-range, beef that was grass-fed and grass-finished, and fish that was wild-caught in waters that are low in Mercury.

In the last two decades my diet has been influenced by many sources and the continual outpouring of new research. These are some of the basics I have learned that I believe have contributed to my health:

- Glyphosate (in Round-Up) and GMO foods are toxic for my body. I try to eat organic food even though the cost is higher. It's cheaper than cancer treatments.
- Processed foods and sugar cause inflammation and are not healthy for anyone.

- Eating a rainbow of vegetables supports good health, especially greens and cruciferous vegetables.
- Eating probiotics such as sauerkraut, kimchi, and kefir helps maintain a diverse and healthy microbiome.
- When I eat might be as important as what I eat. Our bodies need a chance to clean out old damaged cells and that process (called autophagy) can take place only when digestion isn't happening. I allow a minimum of a twelve-hour window without eating (7 p.m. to 7 a.m.). Several times a week I don't eat for an eighteen-hour period. If I finish dinner at 7 p.m., I don't eat again until 1 p.m. the next day. There are many variations of time-restricted eating. The key is to allow some significant time without digestion happening.
- My body doesn't tolerate grains, so I don't eat flour (bread, pasta, and pizza), rice, oatmeal, etc. I don't know if it's actually the grains that are the problem, or the way grains are now harvested in the US with glyphosate. I just know I have diarrhea when I eat grains, even if they have been organically grown. The one exception to this is sourdough bread.

I'm aware that the current research on healthy nutrition is describing principles similar to what Dr. Friesen taught me when I was sixteen. He told me not to eat anything white, like flour and sugar. Most experts now agree that sugar and white flour play a part not only in causing cancer, but also Alzheimer's and many other diseases. David

Perlmutter, MD, wrote *Grain Brain: The Surprising Truth about Wheat, Carbs, and Sugar—Your Brain's Silent Killers*. In his book, he links eating grains with many of our modern diseases involving the brain.

The science on this subject has exploded in the last five years, yet there is still controversy. Some experts say a vegan diet is the only way to heal from cancer. Some people thrive on a vegan diet, while others don't. Some experts say a ketogenic diet is the best way to combat cancer. Or Paleo, or Mediterranean. Some recommend eliminating dairy, or gluten, or soy. And there are "experts" who say grass-fed beef is cancer protective. All sides have studies to back up their claims, plus anecdotal evidence that their recommended diet works.

I think the strongest evidence points to individual differences. Not everyone benefits from the same diet. Somehow, we each need to use a combination of testing, intuition, and trial and error to know what supports the health of our bodies. We each need to be our own personal expert, or find an expert who does testing of our body before recommending a nutritional protocol for us.

There are some things most experts agree on. Whole natural foods are healthier than processed foods. Vegetables are good for us. A diet high in sugar is inflammatory. Organic food is healthier than food laden with pesticides. Michael Pollan, in his book *In Defense of Food: An Eater's Manifesto*, has simplified healthy eating with his statement, "Eat food. Not too much. Mostly plants."

CHAPTER TWENTY-NINE

THE THREE V'S

THE FIRST TIME I USED imagery to improve health was probably in the 1970s. I had a plantar wart on my toe that was surgically removed. It came back in about a month. The doctor said the only treatment was to repeat the surgery. The surgery had been a much more painful process than I'd anticipated and I didn't want to go through it again. I thought there must be an alternative. I had been reading about the use of imagery in healing, so I decided to try it. I had nothing to lose.

I imagined that I had a little jar that said, "Plantar wart remover" on it. There was a liquid in the jar. In my imagination, I dipped a Q-tip into the liquid and put it around the edges of my plantar wart. I did this frequently for about two weeks. When I stopped at a stop light, I did it. When I thought of it during the day, I dabbed a little of the liquid around my plantar wart. After about two weeks, the plantar wart got swollen and red, and after about another week it fell off. It never returned and I can't tell you today which toe it was on. That solid tangible outcome has motivated me to use more imagery.

I hadn't necessarily thought of imagery as a form of meditation. As meditation became not only trendy, but also recommended by health professionals I respected, I thought if I was doing everything in my power to eliminate cancer, I had to include meditation.

The first time I remember hearing someone say meditation had changed his life was about 1972. Bob's fraternity brother, John, a lawyer and definitely a Type A personality, was taking a class in TM (Transcendental Meditation) and said he was so much calmer and happier since he'd started spending only twenty minutes a day practicing his new skill. At that time, I thought, "That's good for John because he obviously needs it. But I'm already a calm person. Not necessary for me."

When meditation became a must in most healing programs, periodically I decided this is the year I'm going to start meditating. Since then, I've taken several meditation classes and the inspiration has usually kept me meditating for a month or two, but I've never felt any noticeable benefit from meditating, so it's never stuck. My son is a meditator and he says looking for the benefit is the wrong approach; he says just do it. But it's hard for me to stay motivated when I don't experience a benefit.

However, there are many kinds of meditation—mantras, breathing techniques, mindfulness focus—and eventually, I found one that worked for me—guided meditation. Although the classes I'd taken taught me how to sit quietly and empty my mind, only guided meditation, or guided imagery, has brought me consistent benefits (like removing the plantar wart). The effect of guided imagery on me is similar to what I'd want from any meditation. When I practice imagery, I spend time getting into a relaxed state. I may listen to music that relaxes me, or I may listen to a recorded guided imagery. Either way, my body goes into a parasympathetic state, which is where healing happens.

I have continued to practice various forms of imagery for the past forty+ years. I frequently listen to guided imagery on CDs, or on digital platforms. Recently, one of my doctors recommended an app called Insight Timer. I downloaded it and discovered it includes 55,000 guided meditations (probably more by now).

I sometimes put imagery in the context of the Three V's—Verbalize, Visualize, and Vitalize. Verbalize is the use of affirmations—making a positive statement about what I want to be true. To visualize is to imagine what I desire is actually happening. This can involve all the senses, not just visual. And to vitalize is to feel the emotion as if it has already happened.

I think the vitalize step is the most important, but it can't happen without the other two. They work best together. For example:

Verbalize: The self-healing mechanism of my body is actively eliminating my cancer.

Visualize: I played a lot of Pac-Man in my past, so the image of Pac-Man going through my body and eating cancer cells is vivid for me. Then I imagine hearing my doctor giving me the results of a PET scan, saying there is No Evidence of Disease.

Vitalize: Feel the excitement, joy, and relief I will feel when I hear those words.

I think the major benefit of using this technique is the effect it has on me in the present. My body is calm; my emotions are happy; my spirit is excited and optimistic. Some people say the emotion is like a magnet to draw that outcome to me. It's possible, but it's hard to know how much this process has affected my healing because I am always using other strategies as well. This was obvious in the plantar wart story because I experienced a tangible change, using only one strategy to remove the wart. It's different with cancer. I have no symptoms, so I don't notice a tangible change. And I'm using many other strategies at the same time.

There was a time when a particular cancer was resolved (words on a PET scan report). I had small tumors on my right lung and ribs, and later they weren't there. Was it the imagery, or the supplements, or my diet, or using my sauna, or mistletoe, or any of the other things I'd tried? There are so many potential factors and I think they all do their part, and together they seem to have made a difference.

There was another time I experienced something tangible that also seemed to be a result of my imagery. In 2012, I spent a week with my friend Patty in her condo on the beach in Cabo San Lucas. We started every morning meditating and using imagery on the patio overlooking the ocean. I wrote this poem following one of those meditations after having an experience that seemed to be directly connected to my meditation and imagery.

Inhale, Exhale

I see the circle of light that has been called
a tumor.
When I exhale,
it gets smaller around the perimeter.
When I inhale,
some of it gets sucked out of the middle,
into a transforming machine
that allows it to become part of the
Courage and
Strength I need
to shine
my light brighter.
Inhale,
Exhale.
I allow this tumor
to gradually be incorporated into my
Strength and
Courage.
It wants to be part of me
But it doesn't want to destroy us.
As I meditate, I feel like I make contact
with a whale.
I ask her to please show herself
I want to see a whale up close.
She says she will if I meet her
Halfway.

This connection with the whale felt so real in my meditation that the next day I went out on a boat to find her. We were approached by five whales that gave us an incredible show, coming up to say "Hello" over and over. The captain said he hadn't seen anything like this for months. I thanked my whale for keeping her part of the bargain.

If that part of the vision produced a physical event, maybe the cancer was being affected as well. I continued to inhale, exhale.

CHAPTER THIRTY

CRYOABLATION

THE STORY OF MY CRYOABLATION is probably the strongest example of the importance of trusting my judgement and intuition and not always following the advice of doctors. I'm the captain of my treatment team and all practitioners on my team are working for me. I definitely need them, but I have to remember that I'm in charge.

The word "metastatic" was first used in describing my cancer in 2011. Metastatic means the cancer has traveled to another site in the body. A CT/PET scan showed a tumor in my right lung. Later, a biopsy identified the tumor as breast cancer that had metastasized to my lungs.

I had always been grateful that my cancer wasn't metastatic. As long as breast cancer stays in the breast, it's not likely to kill me. Once it gets into other organs, the probability of death is expanded. Most everyone agrees metastatic cancer is not curable, but only managed temporarily until it kills the host. The exceptions are spontaneous remissions, which are not explainable in the medical world. Often when someone with metastatic cancer has a remission, the doctor will say he must have made a mistake on the diagnosis. That is easier for him to believe than to believe a metastatic patient could experience a remission.

I felt disappointed and scared the first time I saw or heard the word "metastatic" referring to my cancer. My first reaction to any progression of cancer is usually, "Oh, Shit!" But I don't stay there very long. I remember that I'm a spiritual being on a human path and that everything that happens to me is for the growth of my soul. I just have to deal with what's in front of me. I went into my usual mode of searching for the most effective action to take next.

I'd heard or read somewhere that ablations were now being used to destroy tumors in the lungs. Years before, I'd had an ablation of an extra pathway going to my heart that was making my heart beat twice as many times as normal. Cardiac ablation uses heat or cold energy to create tiny scars to block irregular electrical signals and restore a typical heartbeat. This procedure corrected my heart rhythm problem (arrhythmia). A thin flexible tube (catheter) was inserted into the veins or arteries in my neck and groin and radiofrequency was transmitted through the tubes to destroy the extra pathway. It worked. I never again had the occasional trauma of my heart doubling its beats.

Since an ablation had been a painless and effective procedure for me in the past, this seemed like a possibility for me now. I wanted to learn more. I asked my oncologist about ablations and he knew nothing, so I asked him to refer me for a second opinion. I went to another local oncologist in a different medical system. This doctor had heard of an ablation and said he would present my case to the tumor board in his medical group. I was optimistic and excited until he reported back to me that I was not a candidate for an ablation. He said my tumor was too close to the diaphragm to do an ablation without endangering the diaphragm. He referred me to a surgeon.

I met with the surgeon who described in great detail how he would remove a section of my lungs where the tumor was. It was a major, dangerous surgery that required a minimum of six weeks recovery time. He was ready to schedule the surgery. I was devastated with this option, and knew halfway into this appointment that I wouldn't be going through with this surgery. It would make me into a full-time patient for weeks, and leave me with part of my lung missing. I was sure there had to be a less invasive option.

I had already scheduled attending a conference in Hartford, CT, sponsored by an organization called Healthy Medicine Academy, put on by a group of medical doctors who were studying and performing cutting-edge medical procedures for cancer. The conference was mostly attended by doctors who were open to learning new treatments. I felt privileged to be exposed to such cutting-edge technology.

I also felt the magic of synchronicity when I realized one of the speakers was an ablation specialist from Florida. He had been doing ablations on cancer patients for years. He definitely had the expertise I was looking for and I was in awe listening to him describe exactly what I thought I needed. During a break, I spoke to him about my situation. His response was, "Your diaphragm would be in danger with an ablation based on heat, but there would be no problem with doing a cryoablation (freezing the tumor). They probably said that it couldn't be done because they don't know how to do it. If you go to a doctor with gray hair, he hasn't been trained in this new technology. You need to find a young doctor who has been trained to do an ablation. I could do it for you at my clinic in Florida, but insurance wouldn't cover it."

I was disappointed, confused, yet hopeful. I went home to Sacramento and did more research. I had learned that the professional trained to do this procedure is called an interventional radiologist. I searched the internet and found one in the medical system in Sacramento where my original oncologist was. I asked my doctor for a referral and got an appointment with Dr. Laing. I was both scared and optimistic when I met him. He looked like he was about fifteen years old. He certainly had gone to medical school recently enough to learn the new technologies, but how could someone so young have enough experience to be an expert at this procedure?

He looked at my scans and said I was definitely a candidate for a cryoablation. His explanation of the procedure convinced me that he knew what he was doing, but I still verified that I wasn't the first patient he was doing this on. I don't know how he could have done fifty of them in his young career, but I believed him and scheduled the procedure with confidence.

My friend Carol went with me to the 7 a.m. appointment. He first did a biopsy of the tumor in my lung. They used the CT scan machine to locate the exact spot in the lung and then put a needle through my back into the tumor and took enough tissue to biopsy. That's how we knew it was breast cancer metastasized to the lung, and not metastatic ocular melanoma, or lung cancer.

The area was numbed before putting the long biopsy needle in, and the numbing part was the predominant pain. The scary part was being told all the things that could potentially go wrong. This procedure could collapse my lung and I could wind up in the hospital.

The actual cryoablation procedure wasn't much different than the biopsy, and wasn't as scary since I had essentially gone through it already. Instead of a long biopsy needle, they used a different kind of needle to inject liquid nitrogen into the tumor to freeze it. Since this was being done in my back, I couldn't watch what they were doing. I could hear strange sounds and felt some tugging, but no pain. I felt incredibly anxious during the whole event, waiting for one of those awful side effects. Even though they told me I could cough up blood following the procedure, it was both unpleasant and scary when it happened. My lung didn't collapse. Everything seemed normal and I got to go home the same day.

What they didn't tell me was that I would be in pain for days after the procedure. There was a sharp pain in my lower back that only happened when I lay down, so it interfered with my sleep. I would have to get up and walk around during the night to ease the pain. This was scary, both because it happened in the dark loneliness of night, and because I didn't know if it would last forever. My friend Kerry came over and stayed with me for a few nights which helped a lot. They said the pain was caused by the debris in my lung. It was the frozen tumor rumbling around in there. The pain went away after two weeks as quickly as it had appeared. I don't know what happened to the pieces of the frozen tumor. I just know the tumor no longer showed up on a scan.

That procedure was done in 2012; as of 2021 my scans still showed no tumors in my right lung. I cringe when I think how life would have been different if I had followed my initial medical advice and had part of my lung put in a trash bin somewhere. I'm grateful that I had the courage to follow my intuition, that synchronicity intervened, and that a less invasive alternative was available.

CHAPTER THIRTY-ONE

MISTLETOE

"CAN YOU RECOGNIZE CANCER WHEN you see it, and what will you take out in this surgery?" I asked my surgeon. He had just recommended another surgery after a CT/PET scan had indicated that there was still cancer under my right arm.

After having the lumpectomy on my right breast, changing my diet, leaving Michael, leaving the furniture business, and moving to Sacramento, I had four years with no new cancer. Then in 2006 I felt a lump under my right arm. My surgeon removed this new lump, biopsied it, and said it was cancer. Another "Oh, Shit" reaction. I felt like cold water had been thrown in my face. The next question was whether that lump was the only cancer present in my body, or had it spread? A CT/PET scan revealed more cancer at the site of the surgery. More cold water in my face. My surgeon wanted to schedule another surgery.

I asked him what he would take out. Could he recognize cancer when he saw it? He said he couldn't always, so he would take out a lot of tissue, just to be sure.

I had previously had many similar surgeries under my left arm and knew what problems this kind of surgery could cause—lymphedema, and various other aches and pains. I didn't want to go through that on the right side, too. I asked the surgeon to give me three months to do something else, and then I would have another CT/PET scan. If the cancer was still there, I would consider his surgery. He said, "I will keep you in my heart and on my schedule."

I hadn't been focused on any treatment for four years so I started doing some research into new options. That's when I discovered Dr. Thomas Cowan, an anthroposophical MD from San Francisco, who kept office hours in Sacramento one day a week at the Raphael Center. Anthroposophical medicine was started by Rudolph Steiner, the founder of Waldorf schools. As part of anthroposophical medicine, Rudolph Steiner had discovered the use of mistletoe as a cancer treatment. He observed that the way mistletoe grows in clumps on a host tree looked like cancerous tumors. He created a serum from mistletoe in Germany and found when it was injected subcutaneously into the belly, it strengthened the immune system and supported other treatments.

Mistletoe treatment is now the most studied alternative treatment in the world. A search on the National Cancer Institute website revealed 70,000 research studies on mistletoe. It isn't a stand-alone treatment, but is state-of-the-art-treatment in most European countries in conjunction with other treatments. Most oncologists in the United States don't seem to know about it.

The most common method of delivery of mistletoe treatments is subcutaneous injections into the belly or the thigh. Most patients give themselves the injections. I was nervous about the idea of giving myself injections in the beginning. I didn't think I could stick myself with a needle, but I was wrong. I learned how to take a deep breath in as I'm inserting the needle, and there is very little pain. Occasionally there is a sharp pain and I know I have hit a nerve and I need to inject the needle in a slightly different spot. With practice I learned how to do it without much stress. I'm not saying I enjoyed it, but it wasn't as traumatic as I expected it to be. The dose and frequency of injections was monitored and depended on how my body reacted. The most noticeable reaction was a red spot, heat, and itching at the site of the injection. I would wait for that reaction to resolve before the next injection, usually a day or two. When my body stopped reacting to a particular dose, we would up it to the next level. We started with 1 mg, then up to 5 mg, then 10 mg. The highest dose I have ever done is 50 mg.

Besides mistletoe subcutaneous injections, Dr. Cowan also recommended some dietary additions. I started drinking a cup of bone broth every day, and having some sauerkraut with every meal. This was in addition to the nutritional practice I was already following of no sugar, low carbs, grass-fed meat, and a rainbow of vegetables and fruits. At that time bone broth and sauerkraut weren't as readily available as they are now, so I learned to make them both. They were both tedious and time-consuming. I'm grateful that I can find them at my local Co-op or grocery store now.

After three months of following this protocol, I had another CT scan, and there was no cancer visible. No surgery required. It seemed like a miraculous outcome to me, and I was surprised that my surgeon didn't seem to be interested in what I had done to make such a difference. When he had said he would keep me on his schedule, that indicated to me that he didn't expect whatever else I did to make a difference. Noticeably it had made a difference, *but he never asked what I had done.*

That has been a consistent theme throughout my cancer journey. In the medical notes my doctors write in my chart, they often mention that I refused chemotherapy. But they don't mention anything else I did instead. I think doctors are so steeped in what they've been taught and the effectiveness of what they're doing, that they can't consider other options. If they were open to hearing how other options might be more effective than their treatments, they might have to question their whole practice and what they "know." This step is too big for most of them. In order to continue in their profession, they have to believe what they are doing is the best medicine.

One 'almost' exception was a pathologist who asked his technician to call me when he was analyzing a PET scan in 2015. He said he was comparing it with my previous PET scan and there was a dramatic difference. He couldn't find any evidence in my chart that I was doing any treatment, and he wondered what had made such a difference. All the cancer that had previously been seen in my right lung and ribs was "resolved." He was puzzled how that could have happened without treatment. His assumption was that I must be receiving some treatment that hadn't been noted in my chart. It hadn't occurred to him to give the patient credit for any improvement. His interest was mild, and again, no information ever appeared in my chart.

I should also give credit to my current oncologist who periodically asks me what I'm doing to keep my cancer at bay. But I have never seen any mention of that information in the after-visit summaries she writes.

After firing seven oncologists in the past thirty-one years, I am grateful to have one now that at least understands what a difference nutrition makes, doesn't push unwanted toxic treatments on me, and expresses some interest in what I have learned along the way.

Research is now being done at Johns Hopkins in Baltimore on IV mistletoe. When it's given in an IV, the dose is higher, and the effect can be stronger. I was eager to try it, but it turned out to be a scary experience for me. My Naturopathic Doctor administered the IV a few years ago and within twenty minutes my lips were swollen, my face was red and hot, and I was having an allergic reaction. Of course, we stopped the IV and I was given Benadryl to stop the allergic reaction. My doctor and her colleagues said they had never experienced such a reaction in anyone else. Since it happened to me, I'm afraid to try it again.

I have continued to use mistletoe off and on over the years, and am using it again as I write this. The brand that was formulated by Rudolph Steiner is no longer available in the United States, so I am now using another brand, prescribed by my Naturopathic Doctor and shipped from Uriel Pharmacy in Wisconsin. A book was recently published on the subject—*Mistletoe and the Emerging Future of Integrative Oncology*, by Steven Johnson, DO, and Nasha Winters, ND, FABNO, and other contributing medical doctors. This book, along with the research being done at

Johns Hopkins, will allow the use of mistletoe as a treatment option to grow in popularity as more practitioners learn of its effectiveness.

CHAPTER THIRTY-TWO

ROOT CANAL

BILL RICHARDSON, A SPEAKER AT an integrative cancer conference I attended years ago, said that he had counseled over 1,000 patients with cancer and none of them had recovered as long as they had a root canal in their mouth. Those who had their root canal teeth removed had remissions from cancer. This intrigued me since I'd had a root canal when I was thirteen. Could removing this tooth be a possible strategy for eliminating my cancer? Seemed like a crazy idea.

Once I heard this information, I noticed a little bump in my mouth just behind the tooth with the root canal, and my tongue was constantly compelled to fiddle with it. I couldn't ignore it. Was this a message that this tooth was an issue and something needed to be done about it? Was my body speaking to me? My intuition said yes.

I discovered that dentists and biological dentists have different training, skills, beliefs, and practices. I started researching biological dentists on the internet. Biological dentists base their care and treatment on the premise that everything in the mouth and what happens with your teeth and gums impacts the entire body and its systems.

I discovered several theories about cancer and root canals. Dr. Weston Price, a dentist in the 1930s who researched the relationship between mouth health and general health, believed, based on his personal research, dead teeth that have undergone root canal therapy still harbor incredibly harmful toxins. According to him, these toxins act as a breeding ground for cancer, arthritis, heart disease, and other conditions.

There was another theory that all root canals are foreign objects in the body and they require constant attention from the immune system whether the root canal is infected or not. The tooth needs to be extracted so the immune system can put full attention on eliminating cancer. Made sense to me even though both my oncologist and my dentist didn't subscribe to these theories. It seems like only biological dentists believe root canal teeth are related to cancer and other illnesses.

My research also informed me there is a very specific way root canal teeth should be extracted, so whatever infection might be in them doesn't contaminate the rest of the mouth and body. I began my search to find the right biological dentist who I could trust to do this procedure.

I found two biological dentists who I visited in Northern California where I live. One seemed flakey and untrustworthy; the other was very young and inexperienced. Neither felt right for me. I have friends who have seen a biological dentist in Mexico. I had an email exchange with the Mexican dentist's office, sent him my X-rays, and got an estimate. He wanted to do a whole host of things to my mouth, all in one day, for a cost of over $10,000. It made sense to do everything in one trip to minimize travel, but all of that work in one day would create inflammation in my body and could lead to progression of my cancer. This option felt too traumatic and expensive for me. I continued my search.

I found a biological dentist in Phoenix that sounded sincere, experienced, and articulate in her explanation of how she extracted root canal teeth. After a satisfactory phone conversation with her staff, I made an appointment. The root canal tooth was a top front tooth that would reveal a gaping hole once the tooth was gone. A "flipper" is a temporary tooth that looks like a real tooth and fills the hole. I coordinated with my local dentist who created a flipper before I went to Phoenix, so I would immediately have something to put in the hole and look normal.

My friend, Kerry, agreed to accompany me and provide emotional support on this journey. I felt nervous because a part of me thought this was a crazy idea. I was making an expensive permanent change in my body that might not be necessary, and could be painful. We flew to Phoenix and used the opportunity to visit our favorite restaurant, True Food Kitchen, a chain created by Andrew Weil, MD, one of the fathers of integrative medicine. We have eaten at his restaurants in Denver, Santa Monica, San Diego, Walnut Creek, and now Phoenix. I love a restaurant where I know everything is organic and formulated for both health and taste. Having Kerry with me, and having a special meal at True Food Kitchen made the trip feel like an adventure.

We spent the night in a cheap but comfortable motel, and early the next morning drove our rental car to Dr. Lisa Butler's office. I liked her as much in person as I had on the internet and on the phone. But I was still anxious about the procedure, and wondering if I was doing the right thing. Dr. Butler and her staff put me at ease, being very careful and supportive in everything they did. She deadened the area and I got to be awake during the procedure. The tooth and root came out in one piece without breaking, which is the ideal result. She ground the bone down, cleaned it with ozone water, and put bone graft material in there. Then a barrier and stitches, both of which would dissolve. I didn't have to return to Phoenix.

I couldn't eat before the procedure, so when it was finished, I was hungry. The deadening made my mouth feel full and I talked funny. Fortunately, True Food Kitchen has a delicious variety of organic smoothies that can be ingested without chewing. More adventure.

The flipper fit perfectly, and cosmetically looked great. I put ice on my face a couple of times, and took Ibuprofen. I had prescriptions for Norco and antibiotics (in case of infection), but didn't fill the prescriptions. No need.

My wound healed nicely, but the flipper was driving me crazy. Something else my tongue was compelled to fiddle with. It was a great temporary solution, but not a good long-term one. The standard solution was to build a crown. My local dentist said in order to do this they would have to file down part of the adjacent tooth, removing enamel, to attach the crown. She said removing enamel often required putting a root canal in the adjacent tooth, which was not an option for me.

She researched other alternatives and found a Maryland Bridge, which attaches to the adjacent tooth with a wing glued to the back of the tooth. Maryland bridges do not require adjacent teeth to have their enamel removed. This was a perfect solution for me. After I got my Maryland Bridge, my mouth was a happy camper. There was nothing for my tongue to fiddle with!

Did extracting this root canal tooth have an effect on my cancer? Who knows? My belief is that there will never be one thing that is the "magic pill." I don't think there is one thing that caused my cancer, and one strategy won't eliminate it. I want to do anything I can that may play a role in increasing the health of my body. Because I implement so many strategies, it's hard to know what makes the difference, and I think everything plays a part.

I weighed the pros and cons of having this tooth extracted for a long time. Having this procedure done allowed me to cross one weighty decision off my list. It has increased my peace of mind. I think this in itself has affected my overall health, and thus helped manage my cancer.

CHAPTER THIRTY-THREE

SOCIAL SUPPORT

ONE NIGHT WHILE I WAS walking on a deserted dock in Deer Harbor on Orcas Island, Washington, the only other person on the dock, a woman walking past me, asked if I was Jan Adrian. This was not an unusual experience for me. I often run into people out in the world, sometimes in the most unexpected places, that recognize me from a Healing Journeys conference. They recognize me because they have seen me on stage for two days. I don't recognize them because they were in an audience of hundreds (maybe a thousand).

She was a visiting nurse staying on her boat that was docked there for the night. I was there on vacation. She had attended a conference years before in Seattle and had been inspired by the experience. We were soon hugging, shedding tears, and feeling the joy of a deep connection. Even though I knew this might be a one-time meeting, it gave me a strong feeling of support.

Ashton Applewhite, in her book, *This Chair Rocks: A Manifesto Against Ageism*, said the strongest predictor of long life is having a social support system. Stronger than good health or wealth. This is true for all people, cancer or not. There are many kinds of social support.

In 1989, David Spiegel, MD, professor and Associate

Chair of Psychiatry and Behavioral Sciences at Stanford University School of Medicine, published a study in the journal, *The Lancet*, showing the dramatic benefits of support groups. His study of eighty-six metastatic breast cancer patients found that those women who were randomly assigned to attend support groups for one year experienced less depression and pain and also wound up living eighteen months longer (thirty-seven versus nineteen months) than those who weren't in a support group.

When I read that, of course I wanted to be part of a support group. Although his research was done in 1989, the same year I was diagnosed, it took a few years for support groups to catch on and be offered. I wasn't able to find one for my first few years with cancer, but eventually I did. Over the years, I've participated in several groups.

My support group in Sacramento, where I live now, began meeting in January, 2003, and continued until the pandemic stopped us in March, 2020. We started with a facilitator, but let him go after a couple of years and continued on our own. We had all completed active treatment when we started. The purpose of our group was to not forget the lessons we'd learned from cancer and from the treatments we'd received as we moved forward with our lives. We called our group the "Next Step" group. Sadly, one of our members died of brain cancer in the first year; the other seven of us are alive and well.

Two of us have gone in and out of treatment during our seventeen years together. Even though we haven't talked a lot about cancer, when we do, it's easier to talk about cancer with others who have been there. We can laugh at ourselves and make jokes about cancer that others wouldn't understand. We have gone through many life challenges together—hip replacements, relationship changes, other health issues, and career ups and downs. It's liberating to have a group who knows my history and challenges, and is available to listen to me talk about cancer and its challenges when I need to.

Before moving to Sacramento, I was part of a support group of women in Santa Cruz who were incredibly important to me. That was during the time in my life when I was primarily focused on working in the furniture store. I was working so many hours I didn't really have a social life except with Michael, my husband and business partner. But I knew I needed women, connection, and an avenue for expression. I needed support.

The organization that sponsored this Santa Cruz support group was WomenCARE (Cancer Advocacy Resources and Education), a non-profit that was created by and for women. I was fortunate enough to be a WomenCARE Board member and the support I experienced went even beyond my cancer support group. The women on the Board, and the staff (some of which I participated in hiring) became friends and a major part of my social support system. Without that outlet for meaningful conversation and volunteer work, I might have burned out even more than I did in the furniture store.

The support group provided a safe place where I could talk about my feelings. I expanded my world by listening to others share what was in their hearts. One of the members of this group, Diane, was an artist. I have a sculpture in my bedroom she created. I continue to receive strength from remembering her courage every time I look at the sculpture. Diane, as well as many of the women in this group, has passed on. I have a grateful heart that I am in touch with a few of these women even though this group ended more than twenty years ago.

I have heard people say their experience of a support group was depressing. That hasn't been my experience. I think it depends on the leader and/or the purpose of the group. I have often felt the entire Healing Journeys community was, and still is, my support system. Participants at the conference have told me they expected the conference to be depressing because it was about cancer, but they were pleasantly surprised. On their evaluations they thanked us for the inspiration and hope. The overwhelming takeaway from the conference for both me and the participants was the comfort of knowing we were not alone. Our mission is to support healing, activate hope, and promote thriving. Healing Journeys events never focused on "ain't it awful," but rather addressed the positive steps people could take to improve their lives. We laughed together and we cried together. Talking about cancer and sharing our feelings was normal, accepted, and understood. It was the foundation on which we built a connection. There is a level of empathy and intimacy in a cancer community that I don't experience in everyday life.

In 2007, David Spiegel led a follow-up study to the 1989 study and was unable to confirm his earlier results that had indicated participating in support groups extends the lives of women with metastatic breast cancer. The newest research did, however, confirm that support groups improved quality of life for the participants.

"We didn't confirm earlier observations that group psychotherapy extends overall survival for women with metastatic breast cancer, but we did again show a positive effect on mood and pain," said Spiegel... "I still very much believe this type of therapy is crucial to cancer care."

As with so many of the strategies I've employed, there is no way to confirm that support groups extended *my* life, but I know they've had a positive effect on my mood. That, in itself, could have extended my life. In the nine cancer strategies identified by Dr. Kelly Turner in her book, *Radical Remission*, one of them is having a strong social support system. All of the patients Dr. Turner interviewed who had experienced spontaneous remissions from cancer mentioned support as a factor in their healing. That support could have come from an organized support group, or from the support of friends, relatives, and the community.

I recall the conference speaker who used the analogy of a cancer diagnosis catapulting her onto a second-floor perspective. Before cancer she'd thought the first floor was all there was. Once a cancer diagnosis catapulted her onto a second-floor viewpoint, she could never forget what she'd learned. She could never again live her life as if the first floor was all there was. This metaphor gives me a visual way of understanding why people touched by cancer converse at a different level. They have a different world view.

In my cancer support groups, in a Healing Journeys conference, in a Healing Journeys board meeting, and in a

WomenCARE board meeting, we started from the baseline of all having second-floor perspectives. Not everyone in these groups has been diagnosed with cancer, but they've all been touched by cancer in some way. They may have supported a friend or relative through cancer; they may be therapists who have treated cancer patients. They've had some kind of intimate experience with cancer that has given them a second-floor perspective. There is a deep comfort and freedom in being with people who share the common experience of facing mortality and being transformed in the process.

The women in my cancer support groups, as well as in the Healing Journeys community, have validated many of my feelings, wrapped me in love and support, and given me an outlet for expression. I am grateful for each of the people touched by cancer who have shared their hearts with me in the last thirty+ years.

CHAPTER THIRTY-FOUR

OCULAR MELANOMA: PROTON BEAM RADIATION

I HAD NEVER HEARD OF floaters until I experienced them in 2007. I tried to brush away what looked like little bugs flying around my head, but in reality, there was nothing there. I made an appointment with an eye doctor who said I had not only a torn retina (that caused the floaters), but he also saw a tumor in my left eye. He referred me to an eye tumor specialist at UC Davis Medical Center.

My first appointment at the eye clinic took almost eight hours. A technician dilated and examined my eye; another technician took a multitude of pictures of my dilated eye; the next technician put gel on my eyelid and examined my eye with ultrasound. Between each procedure there was time spent in the waiting room, unable to read because of my dilated eyes. Since this is a teaching hospital, I was also examined by a "fellow" before the eye tumor specialist would see me. It was the "fellow" who did the laser treatment of my torn retina. Eventually, I saw the eye tumor specialist and was diagnosed with ocular melanoma.

There are two recommended treatments for ocular melanoma. One is removal of the eye; the other is proton beam radiation. This is a focused radiation that requires special equipment. At the time, there were five places in the United States where proton beam radiation was offered.

One of those places was the cyclotron on the UC Davis campus, about twenty minutes from where I lived. The cyclotron was one of the earliest types of particle accelerators and requires a physicist to understand and monitor its use. The cyclotron is housed in a huge warehouse-like building and is used mostly for scientific purposes that I can't understand or explain to you. I think treating cancer using a cyclotron was an afterthought and is a minor activity in its usefulness.

I was told the "cure" rate with proton beam radiation was 97 percent. Seemed like a no-brainer and I was so grateful this kind of treatment was in my backyard. I met people in the waiting room at the cyclotron who had traveled across the country to receive the same treatment.

The first step of this treatment was to do surgery on the eye to implant three tiny metal rings around the tumor. This would help them locate it precisely with the radiation, insuring they didn't radiate any part of the eye except the tumor. That step led to the most painful part of the whole process. About a week after that surgery, I woke up with an intense pain in my eye, unable to open it. A friend took me to the Emergency Room at UC Davis and they discovered one of the stitches had come loose and landed in my retina. As soon as the doctor removed the stitch, the pain was gone.

The next step was to make a plaster mask that could be attached to the special chair I would sit in to hold my head absolutely still during the radiation. There was a hole in the mask exposing my eye. Because proton beam radiation is focused so precisely, they can use stronger radiation than is used in other radiation treatments for cancer. That meant they only had to do five treatments, five days in a row.

Jeanne Wallace, PhD, was my nutritionist at the time. Jeanne is a master of research on all studies related to cancer, prevention, and treatment. Her extensive research led to the discovery of a way to maximize the effectiveness of radiation. Immediately after each treatment, I drank a cup of coffee. I'm not usually a coffee drinker, partially because I don't like the taste, and partially because I'm so sensitive to caffeine that I feel internally shaky from a cup of coffee.

Jeanne said that the cells of the body try to reorganize following radiation, and the coffee keeps them disorganized a little longer, giving the radiation more of a chance to work. Even though this sounded a little "woo-woo" to me, I trusted Jeanne's scientific grounding.

For five days, I drove to the UC Davis cyclotron, entered a building that looked like a warehouse or distribution center, and was met by a radiologist and a physicist. My head was put into my mask and I was strapped into a chair. Once they were positive I was in exactly the right position, facing the right angle, and looking in the right direction, they left the area and I was zapped for about five minutes. Then they came back in and set me free. On my way home, I stopped at a drive-through coffee place for my prescribed cup of coffee. The whole procedure was relatively painless except for the shakiness from the coffee.

For ten years, every six months I went through the same eye examination process, meeting with three different technicians interspersed by sitting in the waiting room. Following that, I was examined by a "fellow" (they changed every two years), ending with five minutes with the eye tumor specialist. After that first visit, the process usually took about four hours.

Examining an eye can be an intimate experience. I became comfortable, even friendly, with one of the technicians, and felt a loss when Ellen moved on to another job and wasn't there to do my ultrasound anymore. I had gotten used to looking at a picture of her black and white dog while she put gel on my eye, and now I was staring at a blank bulletin board.

After ten years of going through this process twice a year, I graduated to only once a year. Seems like I'm in that 97 percent who are cured of ocular melanoma.

～

CHAPTER THIRTY-FIVE

PSILOCYBIN

MORE THAN TEN YEARS AGO, before my cancer was metastatic, I heard about a research study using psilocybin with cancer patients. Psilocybin is a naturally-occurring psychedelic compound produced by more than 200 species of fungi. Psilocybin is itself biologically inactive but is quickly converted by the body to psilocin, which has mind-altering effects similar in some aspects to those of LSD and mescaline. In general, the effects include euphoria, visual and mental hallucinations, changes in perception, a distorted sense of time, and perceived spiritual experiences.

Psilocybin mushrooms have been and continue to be used in indigenous New World cultures in religious, divinatory, or spiritual contexts. Reflecting the meaning of the word *entheogen* ("the god within"), the mushrooms are revered as powerful spiritual sacraments that provide access to sacred worlds.

In 1959, the Swiss chemist Albert Hofmann isolated the active principal psilocybin from the mushroom *Psilocybe Mexicana*. Hofmann's employer, Sandoz, marketed and sold pure psilocybin to physicians and clinicians worldwide for use in psychedelic psychotherapy. Although the increasingly restrictive drug laws of the late 1960s curbed scientific research into the effects of psilocybin and other hallucinogens, its popularity as an entheogen (spirituality-enhancing agent) grew in the next decade, owing largely to the increased availability of information on how to cultivate psilocybin mushrooms.

Possession of psilocybin-containing mushrooms has been outlawed in most countries, and psilocybin has been classified as a scheduled drug by many national drug laws. Although these laws have limited the research done on the therapeutic use of psilocybin for decades, there is currently a resurgence of that research. A group of researchers from Johns Hopkins School of Medicine, led by Roland Griffiths, was conducting a study with Stage 4 cancer patients who were given psilocybin in a very controlled setting during which they spent about six hours in a room with a trained therapist. I instantly wanted to be part of the study. I had dabbled in hallucinogens in the 60s and 70s, trying LSD and mescaline, but never psilocybin. I called Johns Hopkins in Baltimore where the study was being conducted and was disappointed that I couldn't be included because my cancer wasn't Stage 4. By the time I was a Stage 4 cancer patient, that study had been completed.

Years later, when I read Michael Pollan's book, *How to Change Your Mind*, I learned more about the resurgence of research on the health benefits of psychedelic medicine. He wrote about the results of the studies with psilocybin and cancer patients. The experience was life-changing for most of them. Many said this was the most powerful spiritual experience they'd ever had, and they no longer feared death. Even though I didn't have a strong fear of death, I wanted a powerful spiritual experience.

I knew from Pollan's book that there were underground therapists taking patients on healing "trips" with psychedelic medicine. How could I find one of these therapists? When I mentioned my desire to some friends at dinner, Joe said the underground therapist that Michael Pollan wrote about in his book, and had experienced psilocybin with, was a friend of his. They were both Buddhists and had been involved in the same Zendo for years. He could possibly introduce me. Even though I have come to expect synchronicities to happen in my life, this one felt like over-the-top Grace personified.

Joe's friends were a married couple. Pollan had done his trip with the husband, and it was the wife that worked with women. They lived off the grid within driving distance of where I lived. Joe introduced us via email and I had an introductory meeting with her at a restaurant in a nearby town.

She was a petite woman with short gray hair and round rosy cheeks. She was warm, sensitive, and wise. I trusted her immediately. She had been leading people on therapeutic psychedelic trips for twenty-five years and was colleagues with some of the well-known people I had read about in the field. We got acquainted over lunch and agreed to do a psilocybin "session" on their property. A session is a three-day event—one day for preparation, one for the trip, and one for assimilation of the experience.

The road to their compound is a dirt road that was impassable with heavy rains so the date we chose had to be postponed several times because of weather. Even without heavy rains, this uncharted road required a four-wheel drive vehicle. Once a viable date finally arrived, she drove down the hill to meet me at a spot where I could safely leave my car for two nights.

There are at least five buildings on their property, which is why I've called it a "compound." Her husband lives in the big house. She lives in a charming one-room yurt, and my room was a similar building about fifty yards from hers. There was another house with a renter, and a one-room building for group ceremonies.

One wall of my room was a floor-to-ceiling window that looked out onto the forest and made it feel like a tree house. There was a wood stove, a small table, several chairs, a mattress on the floor, a high-end sound system, beautiful flowers, art on the wall, and a lightly stocked kitchen. Although there was running water in the kitchen, there was no indoor plumbing. I used the outhouse, which was a few hundred yards away, only for defecating. The entire forest was at my disposal for urinating. My guide said urine is what makes an outhouse smell bad.

I arrived on the property about three in the afternoon. She had asked me to keep track of my dreams leading up to the trip, so we chatted about my dreams and my expectations. When she asked me to write down my expectations and intentions for the trip, I wrote:

What I want from this "trip" is to let go of my ego self and know my Self that is connected to everything. I want to feel my Oneness and know that in this and every moment I am safe and all is well. I would also like clarity about my purpose and my future expression of that purpose.

After sharing a healthy and delicious dinner that she

prepared, we retired early. There was no eating the morning of the trip because of the potential of an upset stomach. I drank a few sips of a liquid that had the psilocybin in it and waited at least thirty minutes before I felt anything. I was lying on a futon on the floor with my guide sitting on the floor by my side. I was blindfolded because the purpose was for me to focus inside instead of on the outside world. Music was carefully selected and the speakers were on the floor close to my head.

My guide sat next to me for the next six hours and wrote down everything she observed, everything I said, and the names of the music pieces played. When I had to pee, she helped me get up and outside to find a tree to hang onto while I relieved myself.

In the 70s, when I experimented with psychedelics, I had the experience of not being able to differentiate between me and "not me." I remember drinking orange juice and not being able to tell where my hand stopped and the container began. I expected to have a similar experience on psilocybin, but I didn't. I was very aware of my body. I felt nauseous much of the time, but didn't vomit. I had profound thoughts and feelings, and felt like my body was a limitation that had to be managed. I thought I could have focused more on the thoughts and feelings if I hadn't felt nauseous or had to pee. When I went outside to pee, my blindfold was removed and I expected the physical world to be different, but it wasn't. It may have been more intense than usual, but it wasn't basically different from the world I see daily.

That evening I wrote down several insights that felt

significant at the time. I had empathized with several important people in my life and could feel the emotions that motivated them to drink too much or embrace Scientology. I really felt the "old soul" aspect of Brian, my son, and understood why he doesn't have a need to partner or have children. He's happy and self-contained by and with himself. I felt gratitude that I was the instrument who had the privilege of bringing him into the world.

I tried to be in touch with my cancer, but the cancer didn't feel like a big deal. I didn't feel like I needed to be cancer-free. I knew I'd be cancer-free when I die. My prayer and intention in this life was (is) to be an instrument, and I knew I could demonstrate that and live a good life with cancer. No need to focus on getting rid of it.

I felt some disappointment after the trip because it hadn't felt like the most powerful spiritual experience I'd ever had. My guide said I was coming from a different starting place than the people who had described their experience that way. I had already experienced the Oneness of everything in my earlier psychedelic adventures, and I went into this experience without a fear of death. If this experience was life-changing for me, it was a subtle change. I'm more understanding of Brian and his lifestyle. I have some understanding of the motivations behind the behavior of some of the people close to me. I had the "aha" moment that "fun" may be the booby prize and isn't what I'm here for.

My guide had told me to pay special attention to my dreams the night of the trip. I had a doozy. I dreamed I was working for a hotel and was promoted to be responsible for the third floor where my job was to be in charge of waking everybody up. I remembered that speaker from my conference, years previously, who'd said she'd been living life on the first floor, thinking that was all there was. Once cancer exposed the second-floor view, she could never again go back to embracing the first-floor perspective.

If my cancer had put me on the second floor, this dream implied the trip had positioned me on the third floor. Another view that I couldn't ignore. And now my job is to wake everybody else up. My guide encouraged me to look at everything in life from that third-floor perspective. I'm not sure what that means much of the time. Occasionally, I feel my oneness with everyone and everything, and I think this must be the third-floor perspective.

At the beginning of the session, my guide read a passage from Rumi to start the day. I didn't understand it at the time, but it felt profound after the "trip" and the dream.

> "If the beloved is everywhere,
> The lover is a veil,
> But when living itself becomes
> The Friend, lovers disappear."

My understanding of that verse now is that when I focus on an external lover as the source of love, that lover is a veil that prevents me from clearly seeing the love that is everywhere. I'm not dependent on any one source to feel loved. The third-floor perspective is that God is within as well as omnipresent and omniscient. God is Love. I am being bathed in love just by being alive. And from the near-death experiences I've read, it sounds like being bathed in love is even more profound after death. If a person really knows and feels that, there can be no fear of death. And any attempt to control life seems useless and futile. In this and every moment I am safe and all is well.

CHAPTER THIRTY-SIX

OTHER TREATMENTS

THERE WERE OTHER STRATEGIES I used that may have made a difference in the progression of my cancer, but wouldn't officially come under the title of treatments. Here are a few.

SAUNA: DETOX HEAVY METALS

My far-infrared sauna uses light to create heat and is the type recommended for me. It's about the size of an old-fashioned telephone booth. The front of it is all glass so when I'm sitting in it, I have a view of the tops of about nine different trees from my second story office window. I didn't know there could be so many different shades of green. I can see clearly how windy it is by looking at the palm tree with the large fronds that wave gently in the wind. Three of the trees have the shapes of Christmas trees, but it would require a helicopter to decorate them. The Crepe Myrtle is the only one with flowers, the color of raspberry ice cream.

When my Naturopathic Doctor tested me for lead and mercury and found I was high in both, at first she recommended chelation. I had just had the Nutrition Genome DNA test (www.nutritiongenome.com) and my Single nucleotide polymorphisms (SNPS) indicated that chelation wasn't the best option for me. My doctor recommended that I purchase a far-infrared sauna to detox from heavy metals. I did copious research to find the best one with low electromagnetic fields (EMFs) since they are reported to be carcinogenic. The cost was $3,000 and not within my budget but when two friends offered to buy it for me, I immediately ordered it from Canada. It arrived on a large pallet in pieces and to my delight and gratitude, another friend put it together for me in my office.

My favorite part of the sauna is the sound system which hooks up to my cell phone via Bluetooth. I can use Spotify to access any music I want. Twenty minutes of Pink Floyd takes me back to the concerts at San Francisco's Cow Palace in the 70s. We could get together in crowds of thousands and be transported to the Dark Side of the Moon, ending with a display of fireworks that held the same wonder that July 4th did for me as a child. I can access a guided meditation from an app on my cell phone (Insight Timer), or listen to Karen Drucker singing, reminding me of all I have to be grateful for and how blessed I am. The sound options are endless.

Of course, the purpose of the sauna is the detoxifying sweat that I can feel running down every inch of my body as I reach the end of my obligatory cancer-fighting twenty minutes.

After two years of sauna use, I was tested again and my mercury and lead levels no longer measured high. I continue to use the sauna sporadically to remove toxins that enter my body on a regular basis just from living in our toxic world.

LISA: MAGIC

In 2007 I thought I would never be able to travel again. I had a pain in my lower left leg that was so painful that I required a cane to walk. When I couldn't find a parking place right in front of my church, I'd drive back home because I simply couldn't walk a block to the church.

I went to many different kinds of body workers who did what they knew how to do, but nothing helped. Eventually an orthopedic surgeon said my right hip was bone on bone and I needed a hip replacement. I did that, but the pain persisted. The surgeon suggested replacing the other hip, so I did that in the following year. When this didn't help either, I felt hopeless and depressed. Both hips replaced and I still couldn't walk without a cane.

One of the physical therapists that came to my home following the second surgery recommended that I go see Lisa, a physical therapist in private practice. She said not to see anyone else in her office; only Lisa could help me. I called Lisa's office every week for eight weeks before I got an appointment.

In my first session Lisa said she worked at all levels and she had to start at the ethereal level. She stood about a foot away from me and waved her hands in the air. Then she put her hands on me and started talking to my body. She would occasionally say "yes" or "thank you" to my body. Lisa said pains in the body hardly ever originate from where the pain is felt. She said the pain in my lower leg was caused by all the trauma that had happened to my left chest area. I'd had a mastectomy, about ten other surgeries to remove cancerous lymph nodes, radiation, and daily injections of interferon or interleukin under my arm for a year. She said that whole area had tightened up so much that there were muscles and ligaments pulling into my lower leg and causing the pain.

For a couple of years, I'd noticed that when I pressed the place that hurt in my lower leg, I had belched. Every practitioner I had gone to said that didn't make sense to them. It made sense to Lisa. She said because of all the trauma, my stomach didn't have space to move like it was supposed to, and the stomach meridian went straight to that painful spot in my lower leg.

Over a period of months, as Lisa worked on my upper body twice a week, the pain in my lower leg gradually lessened until I almost forgot where it had been. When I say, "worked on my body," I mean she held her hands on various places and said, "thank you" and then she'd tell me what organs she'd moved around.

I continue to see Lisa, but it's been on a monthly basis for several years. She can tell me where my pain is by just holding her hands on my shoulders and reading my body. Occasionally she says my immune system isn't detecting my cancer; she holds her hands on my body until she says my cancer is again visible to my immune system. This seems like magic to me, but since she has resolved so many discomforts in my body, I have learned to trust her. Sometimes I wonder if my cancer would have killed me by now if Lisa hadn't shown my immune system where the cancer was.

CANNABIS

In a cancer conference I attended years ago, one of the speakers told stories of people healed from cancer by using marijuana. They were ingesting what I later learned was called Rick Simpson oil. Someone named Rick Simpson had discovered a way of processing cannabis to create an oil that he said had healed him from cancer. I found a source of the oil through a friend and tried it. The goal was to take up to a gram a day, but to start slowly, allowing the body to adjust to the cannabis.

The oil was the texture of tar and I started with just a tad on the end of a toothpick. Even that much made me feel stoned, which wasn't comfortable for me. I gradually increased my dose, but I never got even close to a gram a day. I just couldn't function very well while feeling stoned. During this time, I met a man who claimed that taking Rick Simpson oil had cured his cancer. I learned he had taken a gram a day for three months. He was stoned this whole time and basically couldn't function while his wife took care of him as he devoted those three months to healing.

I also had a good friend with ovarian cancer who followed the same protocol. She, too, had family to take care of her. But when I learned that her cancer took her life, I gave up on trying to ingest the oil. It was expensive, unpleasant to take, and there was no evidence that it was affecting my cancer. I didn't have the resources to continue with this unproven protocol.

I later found a doctor who is a specialist in the use of cannabis for cancer. On his recommendation, I began using an organic tincture that is a 1 THC to 1 CBD formula.

I use only four drops at bedtime and no longer try to keep it in my system during the day.

Since then, I've learned that we all have an endocannabinoid system in our bodies. Some say the endogenous cannabinoid system—named for the plant that led to its discovery—is one of the most important physiologic systems involved in establishing and maintaining human health. Endocannabinoids and their receptors are found throughout the body: in the brain, organs, connective tissues, glands, and immune cells. Keeping this system balanced may be important for overall health, thus playing a part in keeping cancer at bay. There is much research to be done on the use of cannabis for health, but because of the way cannabis is categorized by the United States government, it's illegal nationally. This limits the ability for research on its use as a healing modality for cancer.

I continue to sporadically use a CBD (non psycho-active) tincture during the day and a combo of THC and CBD during the night. I would be more religious about the use if I noticed a clear benefit. When I listen to a lecture that convinces me the cannabis contributes to my health, I'll start using it consistently for a while. As my enthusiasm wanes with time, so does my usage.

Epiloque

PRETZEL

I DON'T KNOW IF PRETZEL rescued me or if I rescued Pretzel. After breaking up with my partner in the beginning of a pandemic, I was suddenly alone. As a cat lover, I had cats most of my life, but had not replaced the last two who died 7 years ago. I had been traveling so much that another cat didn't make sense, but the pandemic changed that. Since I wouldn't be traveling, a new furry friend seemed like a great solution for my loneliness.

I made an appointment at Happy Tails sanctuary, picked out three potential adoptees from their website, and went to meet them. The first one was totally blah. Just lay there while I tried to make contact.

Pretzel was the second one I met. She was in a room with about five other cats. When I went in and sat on a chair, she was on my lap within 2 minutes, wanting to be petted, and purring. No need to meet the third cat.

Her paperwork said she was 9 years old, didn't like children or other pets, and was needy. She sounded perfect for me. But what really sold me was her stunning beauty, her baby blue eyes, and her silky fur. I took her home with me.

She is a very verbal cat. She complained when I put her into a cage, a car, and then a new environment. But I marvel at how adaptable she is. Unless I take the perspective of our souls and imagine that we chose each other before coming into this world, she had no choice about coming home with me.

She is the eleventh cat I've had in my lifetime. We have lived together for almost two years now, and I often tell her she is my favorite. She comes when I call (not a characteristic cat behavior). When she wants me to pay more attention to her, she gently strokes my arm with her little paw. She often sits on my lap and purrs. When I return home after being gone a few hours, she enthusiastically greets me, and gives me someone to come home to. I'm in love.

About six months ago, Pretzel had an open sore on her underside that kept bleeding and didn't heal. The vet called it a mass and recommended surgery. $1,000 later, the vet had removed two masses from the mammary chain, and a biopsy said they were malignant. Breast cancer. She thought she got all the cancer in the surgery, but of course didn't know if other cancer cells were in Pretzel's body. The vet said it usually takes about six months for cancer to progress and I should watch for other lumps or bumps.

The surgery recovery process was very sweet. Pretzel and I bonded. The first two weeks she was caged in a large wire cage to keep her from walking around and exerting herself. At bedtime the first night, when Pretzel was used to being in bed with me, she frantically tried climbing up the side of the cage to get to me. Instead of reading in bed like I usually do, I sat on the floor next to her cage and read out loud to her. It seemed to comfort her and she settled down. This became our nightly routine for those two weeks.

She wore a cone for six weeks to keep her from lick-
ing the surgery site. She hated it. Instead of hiding in a
corner like cats do when they don't feel good, she started
hanging around me even more. Since she couldn't scratch
her head in the cone, she begged me to scratch it as much
as I could tolerate. We bonded even more during those
difficult six weeks.

Eventually her surgery wounds healed, the cone came
off, and we went back to normal.

Then, two weeks ago, Pretzel stopped eating and
clearly didn't feel well. An X-ray showed many tumors in
her chest. Even though we didn't do a biopsy, the vet said
Pretzel had breast cancer, and it had metastasized to her
lungs. This is the same diagnosis I am dealing with. What
are the chances?

Steroids helped Pretzel feel better and eat a little, but
she was no longer her old self. She hung around as close
to me as she could get. I felt I loved her even more. Is that
possible?

The vet said she could send her to an oncologist, but
in her experience, treatment wasn't useful at this point,
and I would put Pretzel through a lot of discomfort. Not
something I would choose for her. I knew our time would
be short.

I have since heard that it isn't uncommon for a pet to
have the same diagnosis as her owner. Some people the-
orize that pets take on the disease to help out an owner
they love. I don't know if I believe that, and there is no
way to prove it one way or the other. But the idea made
me wonder.

What I do know is that my relationship with Pretzel demonstrates the saying I have heard, "If you want to feel love, look for beauty." Every time I look at Pretzel, I see her beauty and my heart is full of love.

Just ten days after starting on the steroids, Pretzel was not eating. She declined rapidly, no longer spending time on my bed with me. She hid out in the guest bedroom where she could be alone. I sat in there with her and watched as she changed positions frequently, seemingly not able to get comfortable.

She was suffering. Her life was in my hands and I needed to help her forward onto her next adventure. It's often referred to as the Rainbow Bridge, or Kitty Heaven.

Although her time in a body was over, I feel her spirit is still with me. For such a small being, her absence left a huge hole in my life. She only weighed 7 pounds, but now that she is gone, my house feels empty.

I am grieving her loss, an indication of the love I feel. Grief and Love are two sides of the same coin. We can't have one without the other. We only grieve what we have loved, and every love will end in loss. I am so grateful for the time we had together and for the love we shared. I am grateful that she chose me.

One way that Pretzel is still helping me is to give me something concrete and immediate to grieve about. In Chinese medicine, grief is related to the lungs. In the eleven years I have had cancer in my lungs, I've wondered if I have grief stored up in my lungs that needs to be expressed. Pretzel's loss leaves me with so many ways to trigger my grief. I can look at pictures of her; I can imagine feeling her furry body in my arms; I can do a rerun of so many precious moments we shared. I am encouraging those moments to happen and consciously spending time expressing my grief. Grief and gratitude intertwined in a beautiful tapestry. Thank you, Pretzel.

STILL COLORING OUTSIDE THE LINES

...But little by little,
as you left their voice behind,
the stars began to burn
through the sheets of clouds,
and there was a new voice
which you slowly
recognized as your own,
that kept you company
as you strode deeper and deeper
into the world,
determined to do
the only thing you could do --
determined to save
the only life that you could save.

~ from *The Journey*, by Mary Oliver

I DIDN'T SET OUT CHOOSING to color outside the lines. And I'm not recommending that you have to color outside the lines for your best life. What I am recommending is that you find a way to determine the best option for you in making choices. When making treatment choices, you may have to slow down the process and not allow yourself to be rushed into a treatment that you haven't evaluated for yourself. One of the gifts of cancer for me was that it forced me to learn to trust my intuition.

When the COVID vaccine was offered, I checked in with my intuition and it didn't feel right for me. Then three of my doctors recommended that I not get the COVID vaccine. They said it could disrupt my immune system and increase my chances of cancer progression. Also, I have had an allergic reaction to an injection in the past. And experience has taught me to trust the self-healing mechanisms of my body more than Big Pharma.

The pressure from the mainstream narrative to get the COVID vaccine was enormous. A vaccine was required to enter many of the venues where I would like to enjoy concerts. It was required to go to a retreat center I have enjoyed annually before COVID. It was required to enter some of the countries I would like to visit. Was I willing to not go to concerts and not travel?

This is a familiar feeling. There are numerous times in my past that I have felt the recommendation of some authority wasn't right for me, that I couldn't color inside the lines someone else had drawn.

- When the lines of the Mennonite womb felt constricting, I eventually had to color outside those lines.

- When it felt right to have a home birth, all the experts said it was dangerous for me to give birth outside of a hospital. I had to overcome the pressure from the authorities to do what felt natural to me.

- In my first marriage, my husband drew the lines of Scientology around our marriage, and I couldn't be me in those boundaries. I had to leave that marriage.

- When I was diagnosed with cancer, the oncologist recommended chemotherapy. The pressure to follow doctor's orders was enormous. But I had learned that my body had self-healing abilities that I could trust. And here I am more than thirty years later, still trusting my body.

- When my second husband drew the lines of Polyamory around that marriage, I tried living within those borders. It wasn't me, and again I had to leave, even though it broke my heart.

It's taken me almost eighty years to figure out that the only way I can color inside the lines is if I draw my own lines. Not getting the COVID vaccine has been one of the most challenging experiences I've had coloring outside the lines. People have put me into boxes I didn't belong in, calling me anti-science and an anti-vaxer. I have learned that judging people based on one decision may not be accurate or fair. I encourage everyone to make decisions about their treatments and their health based on what feels right for them. Coloring outside the lines may be based more on listening to the heart than to the masses, or even to someone who claims to be an expert. I am the ultimate expert on my body. You are the ultimate expert about your body.

If we believe in holistic health, and that we are whole people—mind, body, and soul—we need to consult ourselves at all levels about health decisions. Listen to your heart as well as to your rational mind. It's Both-And again.

WHAT I'M DOING NOW

Death is not extinguishing the light;
it is only putting out the lamp
because the dawn has come.

~ Rabindranath Tagore

FOR THIRTY-THREE YEARS, EVERY TIME I've found out my cancer has progressed, my first reaction has been fear and/or "Oh, Shit!" quickly followed by my research to find the next strategy to hold back the cancer. Now, for the first time, my latest PET scan shows that cancer is in my liver in addition to growing in my lungs. Oh, Shit! This is serious. In my current research I've found a new practitioner I'm hoping to work with who has had much success with treating cancer patients. I've also started acupuncture and am taking Chinese herbs, in addition to Mistletoe and all the supplements recommended by my Naturopathic doctor.

But this time feels different. I'm eighty-years-old now and questioning the strength of my will to live. These last few years have been tough and there isn't a lot of light at the end of the tunnel. There is deep division in our country; democracy itself is in danger; climate change is real; natural disasters are constant, as are mass shootings and wars. And then there is COVID and the fear of COVID that doesn't seem to be going away. Is it worth the effort to continue living in this world?

What if my time is finished? A therapist suggested I might want to consider the wisdom of my body and seriously ask that question. Maybe my body knows it's time for me to move on.

Of course, I know I'm not in charge. My will to live, no matter how strong, isn't going to keep me alive. I've known women with young children whose will to live was over the top, and they've died. I've also known at least one woman who wanted to die and was angry every morning when she woke up and was still here. She eventually died, but it took a long time. She wasn't in charge.

The new practitioner I wanted to work with is Mark Bricca, ND. I heard about him from three different sources, including reading about him in Kelly Turner's recent book, *Radical Hope*. She tells a radical remission story of a high school student who continued to have recurrences of his cancer when he was using only conventional Western medicine treatments. When he transferred his treatment to Dr. Bricca, his cancer went into remission. At the time Dr. Turner was writing the student's story he was graduating from college cancer-free.

When I first requested an appointment with Dr. Bricca, he referred me to someone else, saying his waiting list was long, and there was another Naturopathic doctor in my area that he thought was excellent. I looked at the website of the other doctor, and she didn't feel right to me. I don't know if I was stubborn, or if it was intuition, but I felt Mark Bricca was the practitioner I needed to see. I kept trying and after about a year I got an appointment.

I decided before my first appointment with him that I would do whatever he recommended. Since I felt so strongly that he could help me, I knew I needed to trust his recommendations.

I sent him all my medical records as well as results from recent blood tests and PET scans. In my first appointment with him, which lasted about three hours on Zoom, he introduced his perspective by telling me that he utilized both Western and Alternative medicine, selecting whatever he felt would yield the most benefit. This is Integrative Medicine at its finest and exactly what I thought I wanted, until I heard his recommendation. He gently suggested that I take Ibrance, a pharmaceutical for postmenopausal women with estrogen-positive breast cancer, along with Faslodex (chemical name: fulvestrant), a selective estrogen receptor downregulator (SERD) used alone or in combination with targeted therapy medicines to treat advanced-stage, hormone receptor-positive, HER2-negative breast cancer. He said there was something in one of the reports I had sent him that indicated Ibrance with Faslodex would be an effective treatment for me.

My oncologist had recommended Ibrance for at least a year and I was adamantly against it. The side effects sounded awful. Women on the Facebook chat room who were taking it said they couldn't get off the couch. The TV and radio ads for it listed side effects that ended with "could cause death." Why would anyone want to subject themselves to a remedy that seemed worse than the disease? I cringed at the thought of taking it.

But I had made a promise to myself. I needed to change my attitude about Ibrance if I was going to keep my promise. It wasn't an easy attitude adjustment. I needed to draw on my strengths of open-mindedness and curiosity. I consulted my pendulum (my direct line to my intuition) and it supported my taking Ibrance. Dr. Bricca recommended I start with the lowest dose, combined with supplements he would prescribe to help my body stave off severe side effects.

This definitely seemed like a situation in which I needed to color outside the lines I had drawn around Ibrance. I also had to boost my strength of humility. It was a challenging process, and took some time.

I was gifted a few months to accomplish my change in attitude since we had to work out the finances before I could get it. Even with my insurance kicking in, my cost would be over $3,000 a month. My oncologist helped me apply for financial assistance from Pfizer who makes the drug. Eventually they approved my request and sent Ibrance directly to me at no charge.

I surrendered to taking it. After a few months on Ibrance, my cancer seems to be receding. My cancer marker numbers have been going down, a PET scan indicated some of my tumors are smaller in size, and some of my passion for life is returning.

I am feeling optimistic, but I also know this won't last forever. Often a drug works for a while and then stops for reasons we don't understand.

One of our past conference speakers, Jeremy Geffen, MD, said the essence of healing is "focused intention wrapped in the arms of surrender." I am focusing my intention on healing, and I want to be at peace with either outcome—living or dying, knowing that dying is guaranteed at some point.

Dying is not a failure. It doesn't mean I didn't try hard enough, or wasn't positive enough. It just means I'm going on to the next adventure. I've been told that we didn't want to be born. We were very comfortable in the warm womb, and any other life was an unknown. We didn't have a choice in that transition either and it turned out okay. I'm trusting this next one will too.

Gratitude & Resources

GRATITUDE

Anyone who has published a book, or created a conference, knows that it takes a village to accomplish such a big project.

I am grateful to Terri Tate who instigated this memoir project in her living room. The seed was planted in a story-telling class, and then watered and nourished in a writing workshop. I'm grateful for the members of the writing group that started in that living room and continued to meet regularly on Zoom for two pandemic years. Thank you John, Cindy, Roy, Meridian, Pat, and Lindsay for listening to my stories and giving me feedback and encouragement.

Thank you to the many people who were volunteers and board members for Healing Journeys, always inspiring and encouraging me. A special thank you to the ones still with me after all these years – Nancy McKay, Carol Purin, Fran Haynes, Susan Mazer, Lynne Singer, and Terri Reasoner. Your friendship and support mean the world to me.

A big thank you to Brian Conn, who gave me feedback at many decision points along the way to publishing. Your experience and wisdom smoothed over many potential bumps along the road.

Thank you to my editor, Parthenia Hicks, and the people who read an early copy and made helpful suggestions – Carol Purin, Deb Mac, Bob Conn, Sandra Marinella, Georgia Peach, Lynne Singer, and Kerry Freeman.

Thank you to Flip Caldwell and Karen Richmond for your financial support during the self-publishing process.

The book groups and writing groups I have co-facilitated on Zoom with Sandra Marinella have helped me feel more confident as a writer. I am grateful to the many participants in those groups the past few years for sharing themselves and their writings with me, and encouraging me to write.

Thank you to my Story Catchers group - Gayle Church, Pam Shepard, Sandra Marinella, and Alison Sippel Krill, for your feedback, support, and suggestions.

I couldn't have self-published without the knowledge and direction from Olga Singer.

A special thank you to Georgia Peach and Lynne Singer for your patience during multiple tedious and stellar proofreading rounds. Thank you to Kerry Freeman for walking this path with me and supporting me so generously along the way.

RESOURCES AND SUGGESTED READING

Jean Shinoda Bolen. *Close to the Bone: Life-Threatening Illness and the Search for Meaning*; Scribner, 1996

Alastair J. Cunningham. *Bringing Spirituality into Your Healing Journey*; Key Porter Books Limited, 2002

Jonathan Ellerby. *Inspiration Deficit Disorder: The No-Pill Prescription to End High Stress, Low Energy, and Bad Habits*; Hay House, Inc., 2010

Michael Finkelstein. *Slow Medicine: Hope and Healing for Chronic Illness*; William Morrow Paperbacks, 2015

Jeremy Geffen. *The Journey Through Cancer: Healing and Transforming the Whole Person*; Crown Publishers, 2000

Harold J. Kristal and James M. Haig. *The Nutrition Solution: A Guide to Your Metabolic Type*; North Atlantic Books, 2002

Lawrence LeShan. *Cancer as a Turning Point: A Handbook for People with Cancer, Their Families, and Health Professionals*; The Penguin Group, 1989

Sandra Marinella. *The Story You Need to Tell: Writing to Heal from Trauma, Illness, or Loss*; New World Library, 2017

Dwight L. McKee, Gerald M. Lemole, and Pallav K. Mehta. *After Cancer Care: The Definitive Self-Care Guide to Getting and Staying Well for Patients after Cancer*; Rodale Books, 2015

Mark Nepo. *The Book of Awakening: Having the Life You Want by Being Present to the Life You Have*; Conari Press, 2000

Mark Nepo. *Surviving Storms: Finding the Strength to Meet Adversity*; St. Martin's Publishing Group, 2022

Michael Pollan. *How to Change Your Mind: The New Science of Psychedelics*; Penguin Press, 2018

Sophie Sabbage. *The Cancer Whisperer: Finding Courage, Direction, and the Unlikely Gifts of Cancer*; Plume: An imprint of Penguin Random House, L.L.C., 2017

Terri Tate. *A Crooked Smile: A Memoir*; Sounds True, 2016

Kelly A. Turner. *Radical Remission: Surviving Cancer Against All Odds*; HarperCollins, 2014

Kelly A. Turner with Tracy White. *Radical Hope:10 Key Healing Factors from Exceptional Survivors of Cancer & Other Diseases*; Hay House, 2020

Amy D. Webb. *Stones at the Crossing: Aiming True on My Journey from Scared to Sacred*; Prose Press, 2017

Nasha Winters and Jess Higgins Kelley. *The Metabolic Approach to Cancer: Integrating Deep Nutrition, the Ketogenic Diet, and Nontoxic Bio-Individualized Therapies*; Chelsea Green Publishing, 2017

Nasha Winters and Steven Johnson. *Mistletoe and the Emerging Future of Integrative Oncology*; Portal Books - An Imprint of Steiner Books, 2021

Performance of *Deep Canyon* as recorded at *Cancer as a Turning Point*™ https://www.youtube.com/watch?v=Jv7ZldXPjt0

Performance of *Hero* by Mariah Carey
https://www.youtube.com/watch?v=0IA3ZvCkRkQ

ABOUT THE AUTHOR
JAN ADRIAN, M.S.W.

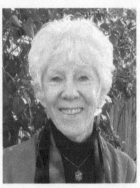

As a survivor of three primary cancers (breast cancer in both breasts and ocular melanoma) and multiple recurrences, Jan has experienced cancer as a chronic disease since 1989. Her background as co-director of the Center for Health Awareness taught her that there is more to healing than chemotherapy, radiation, and surgery. Wanting to help cancer patients/survivors focus on healing the whole person instead of just curing the body, she created the *Cancer as a Turning Point, From Surviving To Thriving*™ conference. She is the founder and director of Healing Journeys, a non-profit formed to produce this conference, which was offered nation-wide free-of-charge to over 25,000 participants for 25 years. Jan continues to thrive in spite of her cancer metastasizing to her lungs in 2011.